Chronic Fatigue

Your Complete Exercise Guide

The Cooper Clinic and Research Institute Fitness Series

Neil F. Gordon, MD, PhD, MPH
The Cooper Institute for Aerobics Research
Dallas, Texas

To my wonderful wife, Tracey, and lovely daughters, Kim and Terri, for their patience, understanding, love, and support.

Library of Congress Cataloging-in-Publication Data

Gordon, Neil F.
    Chronic fatigue : your complete exercise guide / Neil F. Gordon.
      p.   cm. -- (The Cooper Clinic and Research Institute fitness
    series)
    Includes index.
    ISBN 0-87322-393-4
    1. Chronic fatigue syndrome--Exercise therapy. I. Title.
    II. Series.
    RB150.F37G67   1993
    616'.047--dc20   92-6295
                                                       CIP

ISBN: 0-87322-393-4

Copyright © 1993 by Neil F. Gordon

Notice: Exercise and health are matters that vary necessarily between individuals. Readers should speak with their own doctors about their individual needs *before* starting any exercise program. This book is *not* intended as a substitute for the medical advice and supervision of your personal physician. Any application of the recommendations set forth in the following pages is at the reader's discretion and sole risk.

Human Kinetics books are available at special discounts for bulk purchase for sales promotions, premiums, fund-raising, or educational use. Special editions or book excerpts can also be created to specification. For details, contact the Special Sales Manager at Human Kinetics.

Printed in the United States of America

10 9 8 7 6 5 4 3 2 1

Human Kinetics Publishers
Box 5076, Champaign, IL 61825-5076
1-800-747-4457

Europe Office:
Human Kinetics Publishers (Europe) Ltd.
P.O. Box IW14
Leeds LS16 6TR
England
0532-781708

Canada Office:
Human Kinetics Publishers
P.O. Box 2503, Windsor, ON N8Y 4S2
1-800-465-7301 (in Canada only)

Australia Office:
Human Kinetics Publishers
P.O. Box 80
Kingswood 5062
South Australia
374-0433

Contents

Foreword

Each book in The Cooper Clinic and Research Institute Fitness Series covers a special exercise program designed to help Cooper Clinic patients and others around the world recover from a chronic medical disorder. The programs are aimed at people with diabetes, breathing problems, stroke, arthritis, and chronic fatigue syndrome (CFS).

For the purpose of this book, we've chosen to define CFS as "a collection of symptoms or signs, of which persistent unexplained fatigue lasting more than 30 days predominates; or, when no other symptoms are present, CFS is simply a chronic, unexplained fatigue that a person has had for more than 30 days."

I hope you, as one with CFS, aren't so demoralized and depressed about your problem that your motivation to fight back has deserted you. This is a book for highly motivated fighters, people who refuse to let their malady, puzzling and debilitating though it is, get the better of them. They're going to do what needs to be done to muster all their resources and improve their health, though the process may be slow. If you fall into this category, this is the right book for you, for

I feel my staff at The Cooper Aerobics Center* and I have developed one of America's finest—and safest—CFS exercise rehabilitation programs.

Although occasional fatigue is an integral part of life in this stressful era of fast change, frequent or constant feelings of exhaustion for no apparent reason are neither normal nor healthy. Some have hailed chronic fatigue as the mystery malady of the 1990s. Already it affects a sizable segment of the adult population in many countries. Among American adults age 25 to 74, the National Center for Health Statistics estimates that 14.3% of males and 20.4% of females suffer from chronic fatigue.[1] Although many people live with the problem without seeking medical help, more and more worried adults are approaching their doctors for answers. In fact, more than 6 million visits to American doctors per year are now motivated principally by patients' complaints of persistent fatigue. This is a goodly number when you consider that 4.9 million visits are for routine gynecological exams, 5.3 million for dizziness, 8.1 million for chest pain, 8.7 million for headaches, and 16.4 million for sore throats.[2]

Whether a CFS patient is young or old, the disease causes similar hardships. CFS is a debilitator that can trigger a whole host of human relations problems. Indeed, one of the worst things about the condition is its negative effect on people's lives. Even a moderate case of CFS can destroy a person's ability to be productive and fully functional.

Another problem is finding a doctor with adequate knowledge of the CFS puzzle and experience with CFS patients. I certainly understand the anguish and frustration many patients feel when the doctor concludes, "I can't find anything wrong. These tests are normal." I can also understand why anger wells up in others who get the speech "Emotional upheaval can cause a lot of damage to the body, you realize. I suggest you take it easier for awhile, see a psychiatrist, and try to sort things out." Those with the ill fortune to consult a naysaying or unsympathetic physician may end up doctor-shopping. And whether the end result of this unfortunate practice is satisfactory or not, there's one guaranteed outcome—staggering bills.

---

*The Cooper Aerobics Center, founded by Ken Cooper in Dallas in the early 1970s, comprises the Cooper Clinic, a preventive and rehabilitative medicine facility; The Cooper Institute for Aerobics Research, where researchers study the role of exercise and other lifestyle factors in the maintenance of health; the Cooper Wellness Program, which provides a supportive, live-in environment where participants can focus time and attention to the challenging task of making positive lifestyle changes; and the Cooper Fitness Center, a health club in which all members' exercise efforts are supervised by a well-trained staff of health professionals.

Exercise is one of the most inexpensive treatment modalities for CFS on record, yet many doctors fail to recommend it as a rehabilitative option to their CFS patients, nor is it mentioned in most books on the subject. This book is intended to fill that void. What it offers that others do not is comprehensive, state-of-the-art advice on how a chronically fatigued person should go about starting a regular exercise program, including guidelines for determining just how much exertion is enough to improve your overall health without raising the chance of injuries.

Anyone familiar with my books knows that I believe people need lots of incentive to break a bad health habit and replace it with a good one. To motivate you to optimize your health through regular exertion while avoiding the aspects of exercise that are risky for people with CFS, this book comes complete with a Health Points System. It's a great system designed to keep you exercising over the long haul. It will ease you into a healthier lifestyle and inspire you to persevere even on days when you feel tempted to backslide.

I hope this book will serve as a springboard for discussions about exercise between you and your doctor. It will surely make you more self-sufficient and less dependent on your physician to tell you everything you need to know in order to work moderate exercise into your daily routine. On the other hand, you should not regard our advice as a substitute for that of your doctor or any other health care practitioner familiar with your case.

Kenneth H. Cooper, MD, MPH

About the Author

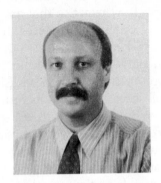

Dr. Neil F. Gordon is widely regarded as a leading medical authority on exercise and health. Before receiving his master's degree in public health from the University of California at Los Angeles in 1989, Dr. Gordon received doctoral degrees in exercise physiology and medicine at the University of the Witwatersrand in Johannesburg, South Africa. He also served as medical director of cardiac rehabilitation and exercise physiology for 6 years at I Military Hospital in Pretoria, South Africa.

Since 1987, Dr. Gordon has been the director of exercise physiology at the internationally renowned Cooper Institute for Aerobics Research in Dallas, Texas. He has also written over 50 papers on exercise and medicine.

Dr. Gordon is a member of the American Heart Association and American Diabetes Association. He is a fellow of the American College of Sports Medicine and the American Association of Cardiovascular and Pulmonary Rehabilitation (AACVPR). He also has served on the board of directors for AACVPR, the Texas Association of Cardiovascular and Pulmonary Rehabilitation, and the American Heart Association (Dallas affiliate).

Preface

Any series of books as comprehensive as The Cooper Clinic and Research Institute Fitness Series is likely to have an interesting story behind it, and this one certainly does. The story began over a decade ago, shortly after I completed my medical training. Because of my keen interest in sports medicine—which was why I went to medical school in the first place—I volunteered to help establish an exercise rehabilitation program for patients with chronic diseases at a major South African hospital. To get the ball rolling, I decided to telephone patients who had recently been treated at the hospital. My very first call planted the seed for writing a series of books that would educate patients with chronic medical conditions about the many benefits of a physically active lifestyle and lead them step-by-step down the road to improved health.

That telephone call was a real eye-opener for me, a relative novice in the field of rehabilitation medicine. The patient, a middle-aged man who had recently suffered a heart attack, bellowed into the phone: "Why are you trying to create more problems for me? Isn't it enough that I've been turned into an invalid for the rest of my life by a heart attack?" Fortunately, I kept my cool and convinced him to give the program a try—after all, what did he have to lose? Within months, he was "miraculously" transformed into a man with a new zest for life. Like the thousands of men and women with chronic disorders with whom I've subsequently worked in South Africa and, more recently, the United

States, he had experienced the numerous physical and psychological benefits of a medically prescribed exercise rehabilitation program.

Today, it's known that a comprehensive exercise rehabilitation program such as the one outlined in this book is an essential component of the state-of-the-art medical care for patients with a variety of chronic conditions. But, despite the many benefits that have continued to unfold through research, such patients are usually no better informed than the previously-mentioned patient was prior to my telephone call in 1981. This book is meant to help fill this void for persons with chronic fatigue syndrome (CFS) by providing you with practical, easy-to-follow information about exercise rehabilitation you may use in collaboration with your doctor.

To accomplish this, I've organized this book as follows. In chapter 1 you'll meet one of our CFS patients whose story will introduce you to some basic truths about CFS, exercise, and rehabilitation. In chapter 2 you'll discover the wonderful benefits of a physically active lifestyle for chronically fatigued persons like you. Toward the end of this chapter, however, I try to temper my obvious enthusiasm for exercise by pointing out some of its potential risks for persons with CFS. In chapter 3 I show you, step by step, how to embark on a sensible exercise rehabilitation program. In chapter 4 you'll learn how to use the Health Points System to determine precisely how much exercise you need in order to optimize your health and fitness—without exerting yourself to the point where exercise may become risky. At the end of this chapter, I give some useful tips for sticking with your exercise program once you get started. Finally, in chapter 5, I provide you with essential safety guidelines. Although exercise is a far more normal state for humans than being sedentary, I want you to keep your risk—however small—as low as possible.

When using the programs in this book, please view them as a draft blueprint and be sure the aims you set for yourself are realistic. It is up to you and your doctor to make changes in this blueprint: that is, to adapt my programs to suit the medical realities of your specific case of CFS. Above all, remember that no book can remove the need for close supervision by a patient's own doctor.

I hope that when you finish reading this book, you'll have new hope for a healthier, longer, more energetic life. If you then act on my advice and adopt a more physically active lifestyle, the many hours spent preparing *Chronic Fatigue: Your Complete Exercise Guide* will have been well worth the effort.

Neil F. Gordon, MD, PhD, MPH

Acknowledgments

To prepare a series of books as comprehensive and complex as this, I have required the assistance and cooperation of many talented people. To adequately acknowledge all would be impossible. However, I would be remiss not to recognize a few special contributions.

Ken Cooper, MD, MPH, chairman and founder of the Cooper Clinic, was of immense assistance in initiating this series. In addition to writing the Introduction and providing many useful suggestions, he continues to serve as an inspiration to me and millions of people around the world.

Larry Gibbons, MD, MPH, medical director of the Cooper Clinic, co-authored with me *The Cooper Clinic Cardiac Rehabilitation Program*. In doing so, he made an invaluable contribution to many of the concepts used in this series, especially the Health Points System.

Jacqueline Thompson, a talented writer based in Staten Island, New York, provided excellent editorial assistance with the first draft of this series. Her contributions and those of Herb Katz, a New York–based literary agent, greatly enhanced the practical value of this series.

Charles Sterling, EdD, executive director of The Cooper Institute for Aerobics Research, provided much needed guidance and support while working on this series, as did John Duncan, PhD; Chris Scott,

MS; Pat Brill, PhD; Kia Vaandrager, MS; Conrad Earnest, MS; and my many other colleagues at The Cooper Aerobics Center.

Stephen Straus, MD, a world-renowned CFS authority from the National Institutes of Health, Bethesda, Maryland, reviewed the first draft of *Chronic Fatigue: Your Complete Exercise Guide* and provided useful suggestions.

My thanks to Rainer Martens, president of Human Kinetics Publishers, without whom this series could not have been published. Rainer, Holly Gilly (my developmental editor), and other staff members at Human Kinetics Publishers did a fantastic job in making this series a reality. It was a pleasurable and gratifying experience to work with them.

A special thanks to the patients who allowed me to tell their stories and to all my patients over the years from whom I have learned so much about exercise and rehabilitation.

To all these people, and the many others far too numerous to list, many thanks for making this book a reality and in so doing benefiting chronically fatigued patients around the world.

Credits

Developmental Editor—Holly Gilly; *Managing Editor*—Moyra Knight; *Assistant Editors*—Valerie Hall, Laura Bofinger; *Copyeditor*—Nancy Talanian; *Proofreader*—Pam Johnson; *Indexer*—Sheila Ary; *Production Director*—Ernie Noa; *Text Design*—Keith Blomberg; *Text Layout*—Sandra Meier, Kathy Fuoss, Tara Welsch; *Cover Design*—Jack Davis; *Factoids*—Doug Burnett; *Technique Drawings*—Tim Offenstein; *Interior Art*—Gretchen Walters; *Printer*—United Graphics

The Cooper Clinic and Research Institute Fitness Series

Arthritis: *Your Complete Exercise Guide*

Breathing Disorders: *Your Complete Exercise Guide*

Chronic Fatigue: *Your Complete Exercise Guide*

Diabetes: *Your Complete Exercise Guide*

Stroke: *Your Complete Exercise Guide*

Chapter 1

Exercise
and Exhaustion
Aren't Synonymous

I t's common to hear a reference to chronic fatigue syndrome, or *CFS* as it's now termed, when watching television or reading a newspaper. What is this seemingly new disease that is tormenting untold millions of men and women around the world and making physicians wring their hands in frustration over its diagnostic challenges?

The best place to begin to answer this question is with this condition's name—chronic fatigue syndrome. It's carefully chosen and, analyzed word for word, quite revealing.

There's nothing particularly controversial about the term *chronic*. According to *Webster's New World Dictionary*, it means "lasting a long time or recurring often." Physicians commonly use 30 days as the boundary in distinguishing acute from chronic ailments.

Fatigue, in this context, is a more elusive concept. Fatigue means weariness, tiredness, exhaustion, listlessness. But fatigue, like beauty, is in the eye of the beholder; one person's experience and definition of it can differ greatly from another's.

From a medical perspective, fatigue is not a disease in itself. It's a symptom, a subjective sensation that a patient voices in the form of a complaint. Fatigue is the perception of being weary even before you start doing anything physically active; of lacking the energy required to accomplish tasks that require sustained physical or mental effort; of having an abnormal degree of tiredness following activities that you've long been accustomed to performing without a second thought.[1] It's only when exhaustion becomes a frequent or constant companion, a way of life as it were, that you can rightfully call it "chronic fatigue."

The word *syndrome* refers to a constellation of potentially related symptoms and signs. In contrast to a symptom, which is a subjective observation about a feeling, a sign is an objective, measurable indicator of disease. Fever, weight change, an inflamed throat, enlarged lymph glands—these are all signs that any doctor can detect easily enough.

When *syndrome* is tacked onto the name of a disease, it implies the jury is still out about it. You can assume that the precise cause of the disease is unknown, that there may in fact be more than one cause, and that not all with the disease respond to a given form of treatment in the same way.[2]

When a new disease like CFS appears on the scene and doesn't yet have an official name or definition, it's almost impossible for scientists to do controlled studies of it. Responding to the need to systemize research approaches to this puzzling new medical conundrum, the Centers for Disease Control (CDC) in Atlanta gave CFS its name and published a definition in 1988 (see Appendix A).[3]

The CDC definition was not intended as a diagnostic tool, but because of the void in hard data about CFS, it's been widely used—and abused—for this purpose. You see, the CDC definition, which lists a number of symptoms and signs that must be present before a person qualifies as having CFS, is so exacting and narrow that it disqualifies many people who probably do indeed have CFS. In the CDC's defense, however, I should explain that its definition is very targeted for a good reason: The list of maladies sharing many of CFS's symptoms is lengthy. The symptoms included in the CDC definition are chronic fatigue of at least 6 months' duration that does not resolve with bed rest and is severe enough to reduce average daily activity to below 50% of the usual level, low-grade fever, sore throat, tender lymph nodes, muscle weakness and discomfort, joint pain, headaches, sleep disturbance, visual problems, mental confusion, and emotional disturbance. These are symptoms also manifested by such disparate diseases as cancer, rheumatoid arthritis, tuberculosis, Lyme disease, depression, and AIDS, to name but a few.

To be sure, diagnosing CFS is a challenge, and it is understandable that doctors have a hard time coping with it. It takes a talented and experienced medical diagnostician to sort out the probabilities from the vague possibilities. I hope you've found one. If you haven't, all I can say is keep trying. CFS is not something a layperson, even a well-read one, is competent to self-diagnose. By attempting to do so, you may overlook some other serious—and potentially curable—disease. I don't want you to use this book to that end.

On the other hand, I realize that many a candidate for a CFS diagnosis has built up anger and frustration with the medical establishment that exceed even the feelings of chronic fatigue. People with CFS symptoms are often told at the end of a series of probing medical tests that everything appears quite normal. They're dismissed with a smile and given a psychiatric referral.

I've been working with patients complaining of unexplained chronic fatigue for years. Some complain only of chronic fatigue with no other tell-tale evidence of CFS. Others have a few of the expected CFS symptoms and signs; still others report the full panoply. Here's the important point: I'm a doctor who advises patients about recovery through exercise, where appropriate. When it comes to unexplained chronic fatigue, the basic exercise rehabilitation principles are similar despite the severity of fatigue and the variation in other symptoms. Thus, for this book I've adopted a far more liberal definition of CFS than the CDC's—my purpose being to allow as many chronically fatigued persons as possible to benefit from exercise. So if your condition fits with the following definition of CFS, read on—this book is for you whether you meet the CDC's criteria or not:

> Chronic fatigue syndrome is a collection of symptoms or signs, of which persistent unexplained fatigue, lasting more than 30 days, predominates; or, when no other symptoms are present, CFS is simply a chronic, unexplained fatigue that a person has had for more than 30 days.

The chronic fatigue that you feel can often be lessened substantially by getting involved in a regular program of moderate exercise. I know because I've seen it work. Indeed, regular exercise at The Cooper Aerobics Center is partly responsible for the gradual recuperation of the woman you're about to meet.

CASE HISTORY OF LISA BLAKE

Lisa Blake is fairly typical of patients whose lives have been radically disrupted by chronic fatigue and many of CFS's other possible symptoms. She's in her early thirties, married with two young children. Besides her family, she has a demanding position as a litigator with a respected Dallas law firm. To say that Lisa is an overachiever is to put it mildly. Before she got CFS, she routinely took on enormous amounts of work and still managed to maintain a normal family and social life. To her credit, she always found a little time for herself, too, sandwiching in two aerobic dance classes each week between her long daytime hours as an attorney and her evening duties at home. Before she got sick, she says, she never needed more than 5 or 6 hours of sleep a night.

Lisa traces the beginning of her problem to a siege of influenza that kept her 6-year-old son out of school for a week. Not long afterward, she came down with what she also thought was the flu, but because she was in the middle of a trial, she dragged herself into the courtroom every day nonetheless. The trial finally ended 10 days later, but her malaise didn't. Exasperated, she went to her family doctor, who gave her some medications to relieve the symptoms and ordered her to stay in bed for 3 days or until she felt better. After a week she still felt strange, but she went back to work anyway.

After a week back at work, in addition to her steady low-grade symptoms, she began to develop what she described as "a bone-tiring fatigue." By the end of each workday, she would drag herself home and have to prevail on her husband to make dinner and put the children to bed. This time the family doctor put her on a 10-day regimen of antibiotics, but nothing changed. A month after the onset of her "flu," she still had the easy fatigability as well as a sore throat, generalized muscle pains, headaches, and swollen lymph nodes in her neck and armpits. But besides her never-ending fatigue, the symptoms that bothered her most were a periodic difficulty in concentrating and eyesight problems when exposed to bright sunlight. She could no longer let the sun flood her desk; instead, she kept her office blinds partially closed most of the time.

The third visit to the family doctor resulted in a battery of tests to rule out some possible causes for her symptoms. When the test results all came back normal, the doctor decided that Lisa must be suffering from a straightforward case of overwork. She should take more time off from work, rest up, and not even think of returning to aerobics classes or getting involved in any strenuous recreational pursuits for a while.

This sent Lisa into a panic. She was an ambitious woman, determined to make partner; a string of sick days on her record wouldn't look good. She had expected her doctor to cure her problem. Instead, she seemed to be getting the runaround. She vacillated between questioning her physician's competence and doubting her own symptoms. In truth, except for her continual tiredness, her other symptoms did come and go, giving her hope for recovery only to have those hopes dashed a few days later when her sore throat or some other ache or pain returned.

All the while Lisa continued to work long hours despite her doctor's orders. However, she suffered for her disobedience over the weekends, each of which became one long sleep-in, to the concern and disgruntlement of her family. At one point, after a confrontation with her husband over what he termed her "self-pitying attitude," Lisa supposed that her problem really might be in her head. She vowed to return to all her old activities, including aerobics classes. But one aerobics class was enough to convince her that her ailments were indeed real. She was so weary from the exercise that she was bedridden for the next 2 days and too exhausted even to turn over in bed.

Three months and two doctors later, Lisa was still dragging herself through the motions of her life with no zest whatsoever. Depression and anxiety added to her burden. Her confidence in her legal ability was shaken. Before, she'd taken on complicated cases with gusto; now she found herself ducking such assignments whenever possible. She felt she was no longer the master of her own small universe. Her life was getting more and more out of control and unmanageable.

At the 6-month point in her travails, Lisa had a job review in which her superior acknowledged her worst fears. Yes, her legal colleagues were aware that something was wrong. Her work showed it, not to mention her uncharacteristic grumpy mien around the office. What was wrong? Given the opening, Lisa talked about her puzzling physical condition. The meeting resulted in a new arrangement: Lisa would work only part-time until she got her problem properly diagnosed and under control.

About this time, Lisa heard about a man who had a litany of complaints almost identical to hers. The difference was that he had been diagnosed as suffering from "chronic fatigue syndrome." Lisa immediately made an appointment with the man's physician, a woman who was becoming something of a specialist with patients suffering from a mysterious lack of energy and quick exhaustion.

With her recent test results in hand for the new doctor's review, Lisa underwent a lengthy examination. Much to Lisa's disappointment, the diagnosis was still equivocal when the doctor finished. The doctor explained that Lisa's symptoms did not quite meet the CDC's strict criteria, mainly because her chronic fatigue had not reduced her average daily activity level by over 50%. However, to this doctor's credit, she also said that whether or not Lisa's condition met the CDC's criteria at the present time was immaterial from a practical standpoint since no one yet knew the cause of this malady anyway. What the experts did know was that CFS wasn't fatal and in many cases eventually went away of its own accord.* Lisa should find solace in the fact that her symptoms, especially the chronic fatigue, were not just figments of her imagination. Moreover, although there is no cure for CFS, her symptoms could be treated and her disability lessened.

The treatment regimen the doctor outlined was long on common sense: Eat right, don't smoke, and, through trial and error, learn to strike the right balance between adequate rest and moderate exercise. Lisa's doctor admitted that "every CFS patient reacts a little differently to exercise," nor can they be relied on to respond uniformly to any course of therapy. Her explanation for the varied reactions was that researchers suspect that CFS has many different causes. The best a concerned doctor can do is monitor a patient's responses closely and fine-tune the treatment program to meet the patient's needs.

Lisa was dubious about the exercise part of her prescription, remembering the repercussions from her last attempt at aerobics, but her doctor insisted. "Inactivity over time fosters rather than alleviates fatigue," she explained. "You'll begin by doing minimal exercise; then gradually, over many months, you'll work your way up to a reasonable amount. No, exercise won't cure you, but it should put you back on the road to recovery. Please try it for awhile even if you're skeptical."

With the doctor's parting words—"trust me"—ringing in her ears, Lisa came to The Cooper Aerobics Center for exercise counseling. A

---

*The results of short-term CFS studies are encouraging. At Brooke Army Medical Center at Fort Sam Houston in Texas, researchers engaged in a 12-month follow-up study in which they compared 102 patients with unexplained fatigue of at least 30 days' duration to healthy people. Both groups had similar records of treatment for other medical problems, clinic visits, hospital admissions, and days spent in the hospital. None of the CFS patients died.[4]

In a more recent study at the University of Washington School of Medicine in Seattle, investigators tracked 21 patients with chronic unexplained fatigue of at least 9 months' duration. Over about a year's time, the frequency of their symptoms' flare-ups decreased, and 57% of the patients either improved or spontaneously recovered. Interestingly, there was no difference in improvement rates between those study participants who met the CDC's strict definition and those who didn't.[5]

Case History, Lisa Blake

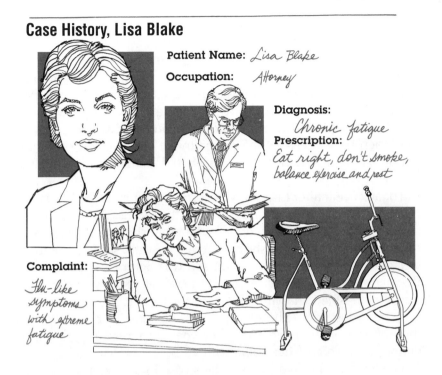

Patient Name: *Lisa Blake*

Occupation: *Attorney*

Diagnosis:
Chronic fatigue
Prescription:
Eat right, don't smoke, balance exercise and rest

Complaint:
Flu-like symptoms with extreme fatigue

treadmill exercise test indicated that Lisa's fitness level was poor for her age and sex, not surprising after her many months of low activity and no formal exercise.

Lisa started exercising in our medically supervised program. Each workout began with stretching, followed by exercises with light, hand-held weights. In Lisa's case, the aerobics portion involved walking and cycling on a stationary bike that worked both her arms and legs. It was apparent that Lisa was a firm believer in the "no pain, no gain" myth, so the first thing I had to do was free her of this destructive notion and slow her down. At first she was limited to only 5 minutes each of easy-paced walking and cycling; then slowly, over 8 weeks, I encouraged her to prolong her workouts until she eventually reached a maximum of 22.5 minutes of each.

Phase two of Lisa's learning process focused on exercise intensity. Over 4 weeks, I transformed her low-intensity workouts into slightly more intense workouts, but the duration never exceeded a total of 45 minutes of walking and cycling.

Our 12-week medically supervised exercise program taught Lisa and her classmates basic exercise principles and techniques, including a new way to view exercise. After she completed the program, Lisa became a regular member of our Cooper Fitness Center and was free to exercise at will.

I wish I could say that exercise was the miracle cure Lisa was seeking; it was not. The important thing was Lisa's I-refuse-to-quit approach to her problem. After 6 months of persistence, her endurance finally reached the point where she was consistently earning between 50 and 100 Health Points. As you'll learn later in this book, this is as much aerobic exercise as she'll need to get each week for the rest of her life in order to derive substantial health benefits with a minimum of risk.

Today, a year after Lisa started exercising regularly, her life is much more to her liking. She's happier, partly because her self-image is more realistic. She now accepts the fact that she may never again be the super-human dynamo she once was. Physically she isn't completely well yet, but she's far better than she was before she came to The Cooper Aerobics Center. A second treadmill exercise test indicates that her fitness level has improved by more than 40%, and her strength is up by almost 50%. She's back at work full time, and she's resumed the housework chores that she'd delegated to a live-in housekeeper during the height of her battle with CFS.

The last time I talked to Lisa, she said, "I see a light at the end of the tunnel. Yes, there are still days when it's obscured, but mostly it grows brighter and brighter. Exercise helps a lot, even just psychologically. It makes me feel I still have willpower and some control over my destiny. I'm doing something constructive for my general health and well-being over the long term. That alone makes me feel wonderful."

CFS: A NEW DISEASE, OR AN OLD ONE WITH A NEW NAME?

Lisa, like most people, considers CFS a mystery disease with a history of only a decade. This may not be true. The medical literature contains evidence that today's CFS could be any number of yesterday's "short-lived" diseases.

Take the strange case of "neurasthenia," a term coined by Dr. George Beard, a nineteenth-century American neurologist and a chronic fatigue victim himself, who wrote a bestselling book called *American Nervousness*.[6] He believed that neurasthenia—literally meaning "lack of nervous force"—was a physical disorder that stemmed from a loss of nerve strength and that afflicted high-strung people who overworked themselves: the classic Type A personality, in other words. Neurasthenia's symptoms were the same as those of CFS. For several years in the late 1800s, Dr. Beard's new disease was the country's most diagnosed malady, but the medical community eventually grew more skeptical, and the whole notion of neurasthenia fell into disrepute.

During the intervening years between the demise of neurasthenia and the recognition of CFS, reports surfaced in various parts of the world of syndromes similar in nature, all characterized by chronic debilitating fatigue.[7] Among the names for these syndromes were *Akureyri disease, postviral syndrome*, and *myalgic encephalomyelitis*, or ME. (The latter is still the dominant name for CFS in Britain, Canada, and some other countries.)

There are differences between some of these other outbreaks and CFS, however. Most of the earlier miniepidemics shared these traits: They were usually confined to small geographic areas, and the symptoms eventually disappeared on their own, often within months. By contrast, the CFS of our time knows no geographic boundary and is usually much more prolonged in duration.

Like almost everything else about CFS, who is at most risk to get it is still a matter of conjecture. Preliminary research indicates that certain segments of the population may be more susceptible than others. Most CFS patients seem to be adults between the ages of 25 and 50. Women are two to three times more likely than men to develop the condition, but recently, cases among men have been on the increase. The vast majority of CFS patients are white, upper-middle class, and well educated; and people in the health service professions are overrepresented. In fact, the preponderance of affluent, young, white professionals with the disease caused the media to brand it the "yuppie flu" and "affluenza."

Further hard scientific data are needed to test the validity of these assertions. Some can be explained away easily by anyone with a passing knowledge of epidemiology and of how a society uses its health care system. Maybe it's an illusion that women are the most common victims: They go to doctors more readily, after all. The reason for the preponderance of white, upper-middle-class victims may be that blacks, especially those in urban ghettos, and poorer people in general have less access to medical treatment, especially for ailments that are vague and chronic rather than urgent and acute. In short, we need to know much, much more.

At this writing, there are several theories—all unproven—about what causes or even contributes to the persistent nature of CFS.

First, there's the *viral* hypothesis. Viruses are minute infectious agents that invade living cells and redirect their hosts' metabolic function to suit their own needs. Once lodged inside a host cell, a virus may replicate itself and release more potent viruses into the bloodstream, triggering either an acute infection that makes you feel very sick or a persistent infection that just makes you feel under the weather for a long time. Or a virus may remain "latent" and do little to upset the usual workings of its host cell for months, even years, only to be reactivated later on. It's also now known that viruses can establish a long-term presence inside living cells, where they can cause slight deviations from the cells' normal functioning without causing visible injury.[8]

There are hundreds of different viruses. The Epstein-Barr virus, named after the researchers who discovered it in 1964, has been implicated in CFS for several reasons. First, many people like Lisa report that their troubles with CFS all started with a flu-like illness that resembles mononucleosis, a disease that is caused by the Epstein-Barr virus but that tends to afflict teenagers, rarely adults. Second, CFS shares many of the symptoms of acute infectious mononucleosis. Third, the Epstein-Barr virus belongs to the herpes family of viruses that tend to trigger recurring illness—the patient gets sick and recovers, but the virus never leaves the body and may become reactivated later. Finally, blood tests of CFS patients often show evidence of previous infection with Epstein-Barr virus. (Bear in mind that more than 90% of the population may also test positive for the same ubiquitous virus.)

Recently, strong doubt has been cast on the role of the Epstein-Barr virus in CFS. Indeed, all that can now be said with certainty is that people with CFS tend to be more prone to viral infections than other people.[9,10]

Another hypothesis focuses on the disease's effect on the body's *immune system*, for which it is sometimes referred to as *chronic fatigue and immune dysfunction syndrome*—or CFIDS. A variety of immunologic abnormalities have been detected in people with CFS, including the allergies that burden a high percentage of CFS patients. (Allergies represent an immune system overreaction to harmless substances in the environment.)[11] Some speculate that CFS could be an allergic response to some as-yet unidentified allergen. Other theories suggest that CFS is an immune system disorder in which either the body works frantically but to little avail to control common viral infections or the immune system remains chronically turned on, fighting intruders long after they've been killed off.[12] Another scenario equates CFS with various "autoimmune" diseases in which the system simply becomes confused and starts attacking normal cells as if they're the enemy.[13]

While the *psychosocial* perspective on the CFS problem is controversial, and many patients resent it, it cannot be completely discounted. It's based on the accepted medical notion that stressful life events and psychological states can have a strong adverse impact on a person's physical health.

The fact that fatigue often accompanies excessive stress, anxiety, and depression is well documented.[14] Studies have also shown a strikingly higher rate of previous and current psychiatric disorders— depression and anxiety in particular—in people with CFS.[15,16,17] However, in my opinion, such data do not support the conclusion that psychological and emotional factors alone cause CFS. Indeed, the cause-effect relationship could be reversed: You could be anxious and depressed because you're sick, not sick because you're anxious and depressed. I think it's more logical to suggest that psychological factors, and the brain chemical imbalances that sometimes trigger them, contribute to the emergence of CFS *in some patients*, but certainly not in all or even most. One might also assume that negative psychosocial factors can predispose a person to CFS by weakening the body's immune system.[18] However, as Dr. Stephen E. Straus puts it, "To say there is a psychiatric component of this illness is not to say it's not real."[19]

Recent studies are constructing another intriguing piece of the puzzle. Investigators have identified a variety of definite organic abnormalities in some CFS patients, including abnormally low blood flow to parts of the brain.[20]

Though these are some of the major hypotheses, by no means have I outlined all of them. There are other theories revolving around genetics, environmental pollutants, an overgrowth of yeast in the intestines, and so on. Considerable research still needs to be done to clarify the situation—especially whether this is one disease (which is unlikely) or several, and whether it or they have one or several organic or psychosocial causes. There is already one highly touted, unifying hypothesis. It postulates that psychosocial stress alters the immune function in genetically susceptible people, predisposing them to chronic viral infections or other environmental factors capable of causing the complex of symptoms known as CFS.

Yes, it's true: Despite the technological advances in the field of medicine in recent years, the cause of CFS is unknown. This isn't surprising. The fact is, we still don't really know the precise cause of many other common chronic diseases—coronary artery disease, high blood pressure, diabetes, and osteoarthritis, to name a few—yet we have been able to devise effective strategies for treating and rehabilitating patients with such conditions, one of which is regular exercise. While regular exercise is by no means a panacea for CFS or for any other chronic disease, it can be an extremely important supplemental therapy. Let's now find out how.

Chapter 2

Benefits and Risks of Exercise to Combat the Exhaustion of CFS

The Greek physician Hippocrates, in the fifth century B.C., first stated the principle implied in the popular dictum "Use it or lose it." He wrote, "All parts of the body which have a function, if used in moderation and exercised in labours in which each is accustomed, become thereby healthy, well-developed and age more slowly. But if unused and left idle, they become liable to disease, defective in growth, and age quickly."[1]

Taking their cue from Hippocrates and other early Greek medical practitioners, doctors through the ages have endorsed exercise as a good health habit. However, it wasn't until the early 1960s that the idea of actually prescribing exercise as though it were a drug to prevent illness and rehabilitate the sick began to take hold. In the case of chronic illnesses whose symptoms include fatigue—heart disease, arthritis, diabetes, and lung disease, for example—this notion that was revolutionary when it was first broached is now considered mainstream.

But though fatigue is very much a symptom of CFS, ironically, the idea of incorporating exercise into CFS rehabilitation is not yet universally accepted. In fact, most CFS patients I've met mistakenly believe that rest, not exercise, should be the pillar of their treatment. Some doctors promote "aggressive rest therapy" (ART) to their CFS patients as the best recuperative approach. ART involves resting all the time.[2]

I belong to the school of medical practitioners who firmly believe that rest therapy alone is definitely not the answer for the majority of CFS patients *once they are no longer suffering from any acute infections.* In fact, I think such an approach makes many patients feel more exhausted and fosters the disintegration of their general health and well-being. Don't get me wrong: I'm not saying that rest should play no role in your rehabilitation. Rather, I'm advocating *an individually tailored, moderate exercise program coupled with appropriate rest.*

EXERCISE BENEFITS
FOR PEOPLE WITH CFS

Let's discuss exercise as a component of your CFS rehabilitation program in terms of the four Ds: death, disability, discomfort (physical and psychological), and dollars. The question you should ask yourself about my approach is this: Is it safe and affordable, and will it help me live longer while preventing discomfort and disability? I think judicious exercise fills this bill for most CFS patients. This chapter explains why.

Exercise Prevents Premature Death

Although there are no definitive long-term studies on CFS, researchers are pretty well convinced that it's not a fatal disease in and of itself. However, if you pay attention to the latest health findings, you know that an inactive lifestyle and low fitness—two traits that characterize many people with CFS—increase a person's chances of developing several potentially fatal chronic diseases, including coronary artery disease, high blood pressure, diabetes, and possibly strokes and cancer.[3] Indeed, our Aerobics Center Longitudinal Study, which tracked more than 13,000 Cooper Clinic patients for an average of 8 years, found that the most unfit men and women were significantly more likely to die from all causes than were the fit ones. In the case of the men, the likelihood was 2.44 times greater and in the women, 3.65 times greater (see Figure 2.1). The bar charts in Figure 2.1 show the results from this 8-year follow-up of 10,224 male and 3,124 female Cooper Clinic patients, all healthy at the beginning of the study even though their aerobic fitness varied from low to high. Note that the death rates soared among the unfit compared to those with

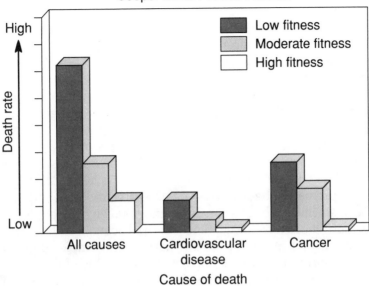

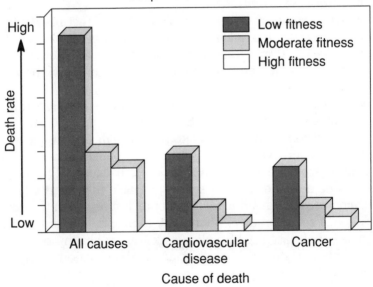

Figure 2.1 Death rates of fit and unfit women and men. *Note.* From "Physical Fitness and All-Cause Mortality. A Prospective Study of Healthy Men and Women" by Steven N. Blair et al., 1989, *Journal of the American Medical Association*, **262**, pp. 2395-2401. Copyright 1989, American Medical Association. Adapted by permission.

moderate and high fitness. The statistics were adjusted for age in order to neutralize age as a factor contributing to a person's death.

You probably know that coronary artery disease, which causes heart attacks, is the leading killer in the United States and most other industrialized nations. It accounts for an estimated 27.5% of the deaths that occur in this country every year.[4]

In 1987, Dr. Kenneth E. Powell and his colleagues from the Centers for Disease Control in Atlanta scrutinized over 40 respected studies that began as early as 1950, in the area of physical activity and coronary artery disease prevention. The group's goal was to assess how, and if, exercise can prevent deaths from heart disease.[5] They came to the conclusion that physical inactivity is just as strong a risk factor for premature heart disease death as the traditional risk factors you hear so much about—cigarette smoking, high blood pressure, and a high cholesterol level. Since the publication of Dr. Powell's overview, several more key studies have been completed and they strongly support the Powell group's conclusion. One of those studies, our Aerobics Center Longitudinal Study, tracked more than 13,000 male and female Cooper Clinic patients. The evidence is quite compelling that regular exercise can reduce the risk, by almost 50%, of dying from heart disease.[6]

Thus, while you may not necessarily die as a direct result of your CFS, it can ease you into a lifestyle that's lethal. People who use their CFS as an excuse to put their feet up and coddle themselves for the remainder of their days are likely to shorten the number of those days considerably.

What makes me so sure that the study findings mentioned above are applicable to people with CFS?

To date, no comprehensive studies have specifically evaluated how exercise can alter, for good or ill, a CFS patient's risk of dying prematurely from heart disease. However, because CFS does not appear to be a fatal disease, it seems probable that heart disease is the leading cause of death in CFS patients, just as it is in the general population. I see no reason, then, why appropriate exercise should not be as beneficial for CFS patients as it is for healthy people. On the other hand, I admit that much scientific investigation still needs to be done in this area.

Exercise Relieves Discomfort and Prevents Disability

With some chronic diseases, it's possible to separate discomfort and disability. With CFS, it's not so easy. The discomfort of unremitting exhaustion and CFS's other physical symptoms pushes many patients into an emotional panic that often results in an overriding feeling of helplessness. This, coupled with the disease's debilitating physical symptoms, transforms people who were once vigorous and involved in life into withdrawn quasi-invalids—certainly a disabling state.

The severity of fatigue CFS patients experience varies widely, as a recent study at Brigham and Women's Hospital in Boston indicates.[7] These researchers studied 40 patients who had severe fatigue lasting for at least 6 months but no other chronic diseases. Besides chronic fatigue, their symptoms included sore throats, muscle pain, and headaches. The investigators probed the degree of the patients' fatigue as well as its frequency. Here are the results:

Degree and frequency of fatigue

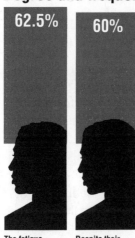
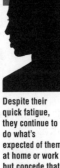
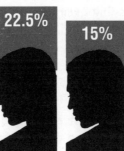
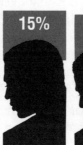
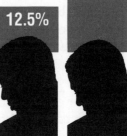

62.5%	60%	22.5%	15%	12.5%	27.5%
The fatigue alternates with periods of feeling normal.	Despite their quick fatigue, they continue to do what's expected of them at home or work but concede that they have no energy left over for anything else.	They feel constant fatigue that may get somewhat better occasionally but is always with them.	They have constant fatigue whose severity doesn't change.	Although they may not stay in bed, they're shut-ins who cannot do even light housework.	They're bedridden and can do virtually nothing.

Of the various symptoms CFS patients experience, fatigue has the greatest impact on functional capability—that is, your ability to perform your usual occupational, recreational, household, and self-care activities. Because the severity of fatigue varies markedly from person to person, so too does its effect on functional capacity—as the following box shows.

THE CLINICAL SPECTRUM OF CFS:
EFFECTS OF CHRONIC FATIGUE
ON FUNCTIONAL CAPACITY

Class 1—Minimal Impairment

You are able to carry on all of your usual self-care, household, occupational, and recreational activities despite feeling more fatigued than usual while doing so or afterwards.

Class 2—Moderate Impairment

You are able to carry on all of your usual self-care activities, but are somewhat limited in your capacity to perform your usual household, occupational, or recreational activities because of undue fatigue.

Class 3—Severe Impairment

You are able to carry on most or all of your usual self-care activities, despite possibly feeling more fatigued during or afterwards, but are markedly limited in your capacity to perform your usual household, occupational, or recreational activities because of undue fatigue.

Class 4—Debilitating Impairment

You are largely or wholly incapacitated—you're bedridden or confined to a wheelchair, and undue fatigue permits little or no self-care.

Class 1 and 2 patients do not satisfy the first major criterion of the CDC's case definition for CFS (see Appendix A). Class 3 and 4 patients may, provided their fatigue is of at least 6 months' duration.

Precisely why CFS patients are so chronically tired is still a mystery, various theories notwithstanding.[8] However, I am one of many who feel that this continual lassitude and resulting disability may actually be worsened in many instances by the very treatment some doctors prescribe—namely, prolonged bed rest.

Please don't misconstrue what I'm saying here. I'm well aware, as you should be, that some well-received studies indicate that physical factors such as muscle fiber and cardiac abnormalities may be partly responsible for the fatigue you feel.[9,10] I do not claim that prolonged bed rest is the sole—or even the major—cause of your lethargy. Furthermore, I recognize that *some* rest can be beneficial: All our exercising CFS patients can probably vouch for this. What I'm emphasizing is that it's an established medical fact that *excessive rest*— particularly the kind that involves lying prone day in and day out—is physically harmful, not to mention boring and demoralizing.

I base this assertion on studies dating back to the 1940s that demonstrate dramatically and unequivocally that bed rest leads to severe deconditioning.[11,12] You may be shocked to learn that in just one week of immobilization, a muscle can lose some 30% of its bulk. In one famous study, active, healthy young men were kept in bed for 3 weeks. End result: In that short time, their *fitness deteriorated to the same extent as could be expected during 30 years of normal aging!* The specific negative effects of immobility include

- atrophy (wasting) and weakness of the muscles, tendons, and ligaments;
- reduction in the pumping ability of the heart muscle;
- impairment of normal lung function and an increased predisposition for lung collapse and pneumonia;
- an excessive rise in the heart rate and fall in systolic blood pressure, merely from shifting positions;
- an increased risk of blood clots;
- greater risk of breaking a bone due to the loss of bone mass, or osteoporosis; and
- far more joint stiffness and much less range of joint motion.

Given these indisputable facts about bed rest, I find it paradoxical when doctors respond to their patients' complaints about weakness and fatigue by recommending even more rest. Their "prescription" sets in motion a vicious cycle of more rest leading to more fatigue.[13]

Yes, some of your fatigue probably results from an underlying and still unexplained disease process. But I suggest that your fatigue is also partly caused by simple inactivity. Look at it this way: That excessive rest you're engaging in may be making you feel 30 years older.

Regular exercise is crucial because it boosts fitness. And it can boost fitness in almost anyone, even in patients with other chronic diseases more serious from a fatality standpoint than CFS. Regular exercise sets up a beneficial cycle that spirals upward and works this way: The fitter you are, the longer and more strenuously you can exert yourself before exhaustion overtakes you. The longer and the more intensely you exercise—within the limits I discuss later in this book—the more your fitness will improve over time.

While no studies focusing solely on CFS patients' ability to increase their fitness level with exercise have yet been undertaken, three investigations shed some light on the subject.

The first study was conducted in Sweden in the 1950s.[14] It involved eight patients with *vasoregulatory asthenia*, a disorder accompanied by chronic fatigue and thought to be closely related to CFS. After undergoing unsuccessful therapy with a variety of medications, the patients participated in 6 weeks of muscle-strengthening and aerobic exercise training. *On completion of training, fitness levels had increased by an average of 58% in the two male study participants and by an amazing 100% in the six female study participants.* Before training, two patients were incapable of performing occupational work, and none could perform full-time work without experiencing various symptoms. After training, none were completely incapacitated, and three performed full-time work free of symptoms. Impressive findings, indeed.

The second study involved 382 Cooper Clinic patients ages 30 to 65.[15] All were given a comprehensive preventive medical exam and put through a treadmill exercise test, which found them to be unfit. Though none had any major chronic diseases, 43 complained of chronic fatigue. All got the same advice: Increase your level of physical activity.

When they were reevaluated about 2-1/2 years later, we paid special attention to those who had initially reported fatigue, and found that 44% of them had substantially increased their fitness level. Of the nonfatigued study participants, 45% had substantially increased their fitness level. Note that the two percentages are almost identical.

Here's the part that will probably interest you most: *Of the chronic fatigue patients with heightened fitness levels, more than two-thirds said that their earlier exhaustion had disappeared.* Only 46% of those whose fitness levels hadn't changed said that their exhaustion problems had disappeared.

These results suggest two things: First, many CFS patients can attain fitness improvements similar to those of healthy people. Second, regular exercise can help alleviate chronic fatigue in many cases.

A final study of note took place at the University of Western Ontario in Canada and involved 42 patients with *fibromyalgia*, of which a distinguishing symptom is chronic fatigue. Fibromyalgia is a disease of unknown origin that is characterized by widespread musculoskeletal pain, tenderness at many specific sites on the body, and other symptoms, including persistent tiredness. Because many patients with CFS meet the diagnostic criteria for fibromyalgia and vice versa, some experts think the two diseases may have similar causes and may respond to similar treatments.[16]

The participants were divided into two groups. Of those who engaged in 20 weeks of strenuous aerobic exercise, *83% increased their fitness by 25% or more*; none of the nonexercisers did. The exercising patients also decreased the overall severity of their disease, improved their mental outlook, and reported less muscle pain. None complained that exercise triggered any troubling side effects.[17]

Exercise Alleviates
CFS's Psychological Distress

CFS forces many people to change their lifestyles, not to mention worry about the future in general and how to pay medical bills in particular. The emotional pain such changes trigger can be just as hard to deal with as physical pain and discomfort.

Although I'd be foolish to claim that regular exercise is a panacea for psychological problems, I do know it can help profoundly, based on scientific as well as anecdotal evidence. Several studies have concluded that chronic disease patients who are faithful exercisers suffer less from stress, anxiety, and depression; they sleep better and have an enhanced sense of self-esteem.[18] A consensus panel of the National Institute of Mental Health in the United States likewise maintains that exercise and physical fitness have a positive influence on most people's mental outlook and well-being, no matter what their age. Regular exercise helps control stress, reduce anxiety, and relieve depression. While major depression requires medication and psychotherapy, exercise is seen as a useful adjunct to them.[19]

How does exercise enhance self-esteem? It's well known in the exercise community that about half of all people who start an aerobics exercise program drop out by the third to sixth month. If you can defy this statistic, imagine how you'll feel. In effect, exercise will come to symbolize your perseverance, your ability to make a commitment to something and stick with it through thick and thin. Exercise will provide tangible proof that you really do have more control than you thought over your condition. This knowledge will help prevent a syndrome known as *learned helplessness*, in which patients come to believe their affliction is totally beyond their control, and must be borne with as much stoicism as possible. Learned helplessness results in a vicious downward spiral of further psychological problems and dependence on others. Taken to its logical conclusion, invalidism is the end result.

Ken Cooper likes to tout exercise as "nature's own tranquilizer." He and others believe that this tranquilizing effect occurs in part because aerobic exercise triggers the release of endorphins, hormones produced by the pituitary gland in the brain. Once endorphins enter the bloodstream, their beneficial effects are thought to last several hours. Those effects are two-fold. The first is some relief from any pain that may accompany your CFS; the second is a sense of euphoria, a feeling that all is right with the world.[20]

Exercise Provides Dollar Advantages

CFS can be an expensive disease, not necessarily in dollars spent for medical treatment, but in dollars lost while you're too disabled to work. If exercise can improve your fitness and functional capacity, it's also likely to enhance your productivity. With some luck and perseverance this should translate directly into dollars earned.

I don't want to leave you with the impression that participating in an exercise program is free of expense. As a CFS patient, you'll incur the cost of periodic medical evaluations and testing. In the beginning, you may have fees for participating in a supervised exercise program or joining a health club. You might want to purchase exercise equipment. Such expenses can be kept to a minimum. The first one—periodic medical checkups—is the only expense that the average exercising CFS patient can't do without. But, for those of you with mild or moderate CFS, the cost of a medical screening before you begin your program and the price of a good pair of walking shoes may be the extent of your financial outlay.

By now you should be convinced that regular exercise has many potential benefits for persons with CFS. However, please keep in mind that, to be most effective, regular exercise must be combined with appropriate medical care and positive changes in lifestyle, such as correct nutrition and quitting smoking.

RISKS FROM EXERCISE

Yes, there are some. The major health hazards for anyone engaging in *vigorous* exercise are musculoskeletal injuries and cardiac complications. For people with CFS, there's the additional risk that the wrong kind of exercise, or too much of it, could worsen their condition.

Musculoskeletal Injuries

Even healthy adults who exercise occasionally suffer musculoskeletal injuries. Two recent studies estimate that some 50% of all competitive runners sustain at least 1 exercise-related injury each year.[21,22] However, these are serious amateur or professional runners. When the sample involves only recreational exercisers, the story is much different. Such studies, including one conducted at The Cooper Institute for Aerobics Research,[23] suggest that the number of exercise-induced injuries among noncompetitive athletes is not nearly as high as commonly believed. It's estimated that musculoskeletal injuries serious enough to require medical care probably occur at an annual rate of less than 5% among recreational exercisers. In chapter 5 I tell you how to take precautions to minimize your risk for musculoskeletal injuries.

Cardiac Complications

We've all read or heard about people who drop dead suddenly from a heart attack while exercising. It's a chilling picture that might make you wonder if it's safe to exercise.

Studies make it clear that exercise itself is not the problem.[24] It's the lethal combination of injudicious, vigorous exertion and preexisting coronary artery disease that you may not know you have. In chapter 5 I'll tell you how to determine whether you have coronary artery disease and, if you do, how to minimize your risk of a potentially fatal cardiac event during exercise. Be assured that when appropriate precautions are taken exercise is exceptionally safe even for most people with heart disease.

In addition to coronary artery disease, one other cardiac disorder may be of concern to some with CFS. It's well known that acute viral infections such as influenza tend to attack muscle cells throughout the body; your heart is one of those muscles. Evidence suggests that 2% to 5% of influenza patients generally experience some degree of cardiac involvement. During some influenza epidemics, these estimates can soar to 12%.[25] A viral infection of the heart muscle cells can cause an inflammatory condition known as *viral myocarditis*. Fortunately, it's usually mild, has no symptoms, and disappears of its own accord. When it does turn serious, though, irreversible heart damage can result; on rare occasions it can be fatal.

What has this got to do with CFS and exercise?

A persistent viral infection is one possible cause of CFS. It's also been suggested, though there's no proof, that some CFS patients suffer from latent viral infections of the heart muscle cells.[26] Moreover, studies conducted in mice with certain acute viral infections show that strenuous exercise can both predispose them to, and exacerbate, the severity of viral myocarditis.[27,28] Thus, it can be concluded that vigorous exercise could make some CFS patients more susceptible to viral myocarditis.

Before you shut this book and throw away your walking shoes, let me explain why I and many infectious disease experts believe that it's safe for most CFS patients to exercise, provided you take proper precautions. There's a distinction between *acute* and *chronic* viral infections. When you have an acute infection, such as influenza, you're sick and you usually know it. A chronic viral infection, like some CFS patients have, wears you down, but it doesn't necessarily lay you up and put you totally out of commission. It's acute rather than chronic viral infections that have been known to trigger viral myocarditis when combined with strenuous exertion. To date there have been no reports of viral myocarditis developing in people with CFS who exercise. Indeed, in the population as a whole, viral myocarditis is a very rare cause of death and an even rarer cause of sudden death during exercise.

I wish there were a greater body of research studies on CFS I could comb for more definitive answers on the issue of exercise and the risk for viral myocarditis. However, there are several studies worth mentioning. These studies probed the effect of exercise training on patients recovering from classic viral infections. No study that I know of has concluded that exercise had an adverse influence.[29] To the contrary, in a 1964 study of 131 Harvard University students with infectious mononucleosis, those who were confined to bed actually recovered more slowly than those who were encouraged to maintain their usual activity schedules.[30] Mononucleosis is caused by the Epstein-Barr virus, which, as you know, is one of the viruses that's suspected of causing CFS.

More recently, Dr. Harvey B. Simon from the Cardiovascular Health Center and Infectious Disease Unit of Harvard Medical School and Massachusetts General Hospital reviewed all the available literature and concluded that "bed rest has been prescribed much more often than is necessary in patients with [viral] hepatitis and mono-nucleosis."[31]

I believe the same observation may be made about CFS. Yes, CFS patients with a fever or other symptoms pointing to an acute viral infection should avoid strenuous exercise. But there is no evidence that CFS patients without such active symptoms or measurable signs should restrict appropriately performed exercise, especially out of a fear that exertion will precipitate viral myocarditis.

Worsening of CFS

You're probably aware that some experts maintain that any exercise will make CFS patients worse and may even speed up the progression of the disease.[32]

I've already provided you with evidence that exercise can, in fact, be beneficial *as long as you ease into it gradually and take appropriate precautions.* If you do too much too soon, you'll surely feel worse. It's a common mistake that people beginning an exercise program make. Even healthy people who start an exercise program like gangbusters do themselves more harm than good and end up feeling exhausted.

What about the possibility that exercise may aggravate the as-yet unknown factors that cause CFS?

Two of the prime culprits suspected as causative agents, chronic viral infections and psychological disorders, are probably not adversely affected by exercise, as I've already pointed out. In fact, when it comes to psychological disorders, exercise, if anything, tends to help alleviate such maladies.

A third suspected causative agent is a disorder of the immune system. I've reviewed the existing studies on the relationship between exercise and the immune system and found that *appropriate exercise* doesn't appear to have a detrimental effect on the immune system; it may even be beneficial. On the other hand, *excessive exercise* can, indeed, pose problems.[33]

You must make the distinction between appropriate exercise and excessive exercise. Indeed, it would be accurate to view exercise as a two-edged sword. Used properly, there's little doubt that it can help you win the battle against CFS. Used injudiciously, however, it can become a weapon in the camp of the enemy—that onerous, mystifying disease that's slowly eating away at your physical stamina, not to mention your peace of mind.

The point I always impress upon CFS patients is that things have changed. What once seemed easy for you in the way of exercise may now represent overexertion. You must deal with your body in its present state. Do not compare the current you with the old you.

Balance of appropriate vs. excessive exercise

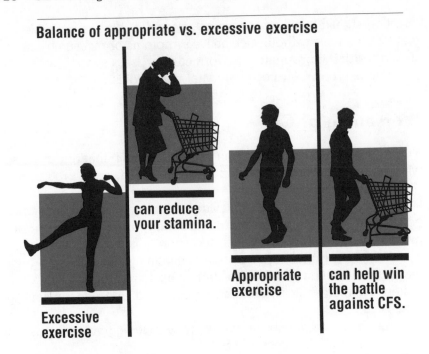

can reduce
your stamina.

Appropriate
exercise

can help win
the battle
against CFS.

Excessive
exercise

Forget past glories on the football field or the tennis court and face what's happening with your body now.

Chapter 2

Prescription

☐ Include exercise in your CFS treatment/rehabilitation program.
☐ Exercise regularly to reduce your risk for premature death.
☐ Exercise regularly to help relieve your fatigue and minimize your long-term disability.
☐ Exercise regularly to alleviate psychological distress.
☐ Exercise regularly to enhance your productivity and thereby re-duce the economic burden of your CFS.
☐ Keep in mind that exercise is not a panacea, but rather an extremely important supplemental therapy.
☐ To gain optimal benefits, combine regular exercise with appro-priate medical care and other positive lifestyle changes.
☐ Be aware that inappropriate exercise could worsen your CFS and any complications stemming from it.
☐ Obtain your doctor's consent before embarking on an exercise program.

Chapter 3

Getting Started on a Regular Exercise Program

I'd like you to approach exercise as a form of CFS medication. Since exercise makes people tired, this may strike you as paradoxical. In truth, exercise, especially if it's moderate, only makes people tired momentarily. Soon thereafter, they feel refreshed. And if they exercise regularly, their energy level increases and fatigue decreases.

Because of your malady, it may take you a little longer than the average person to start enjoying exercise. But with a little perseverance, I think you'll soon see why exercise should be an integral part of your rehabilitation program.

COMPONENTS OF AN EXERCISE WORKOUT

In a typical exercise session you should spend 10 to 20 minutes doing stretching and muscle-strengthening exercises. The next 5 minutes should be spent in an aerobic warm-up, followed by 15 to 60 minutes of aerobic exercise at an appropriate intensity. Spend 5 minutes cooling down aerobically, and finish your session with 5 minutes of stretching exercises. You'll note that stretching and muscle strengthening are included at the beginning, and stretching exercises are repeated at the end of the workout. Please keep in mind that it may take you several weeks to gradually work your way up to the durations I've specified for certain components.

Time spent in workout activities

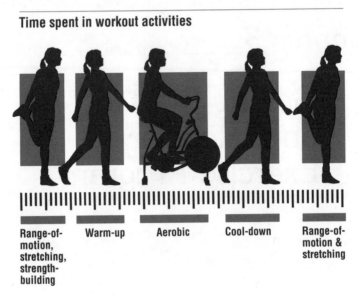

| Range-of-motion, stretching, strength-building | Warm-up | Aerobic | Cool-down | Range-of-motion & stretching |

What's the rationale for doing all these forms of exercise?

Granted, the aerobic portion of the workout is the most important component because it is meant to increase your fitness, reduce your fatigue and certain other CFS symptoms, and lower your risk for other chronic conditions, heart disease in particular. But stretching and strengthening your muscles shouldn't be overlooked either. After all, without well-functioning muscles, you wouldn't be able to undertake aerobics and many other recreational, occupational, and self-care activities. Also, weak, stiff, inflexible muscles can undoubtedly exacerbate your fatigue and increase the likelihood of musculoskeletal injuries. Indeed, these two components of a balanced exercise program are so important that I am currently engaged in a 5-year research study, funded by the National Institutes of Health, to document their health benefits; and The Cooper Institute for Aerobics Research's book, *The Strength Connection*, deals almost exclusively with strength training.[1]

Stretching Exercises

Stretching is part of a good exercise regimen. It should always precede an aerobic exercise session, whether or not you have CFS. It won't take you long to appreciate the value of stretching: It relaxes you mentally and physically, and it probably helps reduce chronic fatigue and prevent injuries by increasing your flexibility and widening your freedom of movement.

At the beginning of an exercise session, and at the end, if you have time (and I encourage you to make time), do several of the stretches described and shown in Figures 3.1 through 3.5. Over the years, I have found these to be particularly useful.

Basic Guidelines for Stretching Exercises

Before and after each aerobic exercise session, do 1-3 repetitions of each stretching exercise shown here. Each stretch should be held for 10-20 seconds with no bouncing movements. Do not stretch to the point where the exercise becomes painful. Remember to keep breathing regularly—do not hold your breath.

If you've had previous joint surgery or suffer from any musculo-skeletal problems such as arthritis, be sure to check with your doctor before doing these exercises.

Shoulder and Back Stretch. Lift your right elbow toward the ceiling and place your right hand as far down your back as possible between the shoulder blades. Allow your chin to rest on your chest. If possible, using your left hand, gently pull your right elbow to the left until a stretch is felt on the back of the right arm and down the right side of the back. Hold. Repeat with the left arm.

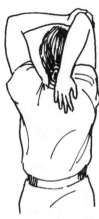

Figure 3.1

Inner Thigh Stretch. Sit on the floor, place the soles of your feet together, and pull your heels in as close to the buttocks as possible. Gently press your knees down toward the floor.

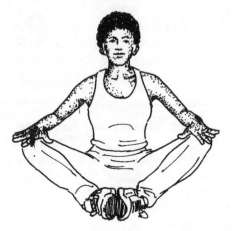

Figure 3.2

Lower Back and Hamstring Stretch. Sit on the floor with your legs straight out in front of you and your hands on your thighs. Bend forward slowly, reaching toward your toes. Keep your head and back aligned as you move into the stretch. If necessary, you can slightly bend your knees.

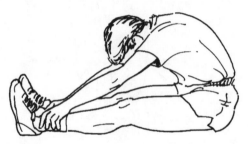

Figure 3.3

Lower Back, Thigh, and Hip Stretch. Lie flat on your back with your legs extended on the floor. Pull your right knee up to your chest and press your back to the floor. Hold this position and then repeat with the left knee.

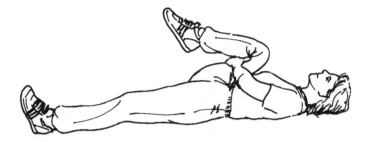

Figure 3.4

Calf Stretch. Stand facing a wall, approximately 3 feet away. Place your palms on the wall, keeping your feet flat on the floor. Leave one foot in place as you step forward with the other. Make sure your back remains straight as you gently bend the front knee forward toward the wall. Repeat the same exercise with the opposite leg.

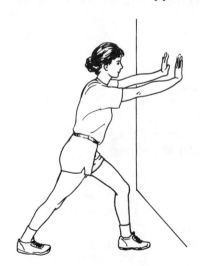

Figure 3.5

Muscle-Strengthening Exercises

Unlike flexibility training, which you should include in all your workouts (usually 3 to 5 days each week), muscle-strengthening exercises need to be done only 2 or 3 days a week—and *not* on consecutive days. These exercises can be done either before or after the aerobic portion of your workout.

The American College of Sports Medicine recommends that the average healthy adult perform at least 2 times a week a minimum of 8 to 10 exercises involving the major muscle groups. They further urge adults to perform at least one set, consisting of 8 to 12 repetitions, of each strength-building exercise during each muscle-strengthening workout.[2] These recommendations are appropriate for people with CFS. However, if you've got both CFS and heart disease, I suggest you consult *The Cooper Clinic Cardiac Rehabilitation Program*[3] for more extensive guidelines.

The program that follows works all the major muscles of the body and requires the use of light hand-held weights, ranging from a beginning weight of 1 to 6 pounds (about 0.5 to 3 kilograms), to a top weight of 13 pounds (about 6 kilograms). If you wish to exceed 13 pounds, consider the severity of your CFS and whether you have any other chronic diseases. If you do, consult your doctor before proceeding.

If your doctor clears you to undertake a more strenuous strength-building program than the one described and shown in Figures 3.6 to 3.16, I encourage you to find an adequately trained health professional who is familiar with your case and willing to instruct you in the correct use of strength-training equipment. A well-equipped gym might be outfitted with weight-training devices carrying such brand names as Cybex Strength Systems, Hydrafitness, Nautilus, and Universal. These are excellent machines provided that someone carefully instructs you how to use them and supervises your exercise.

Muscle-Strengthening Exercises Using Hand-Held Weights

These are strength-building routines that most people with CFS can do at home with little risk of adverse consequences. Nevertheless, I suggest that you discuss my program with your doctor and get his or her okay to proceed.

I recommend that you perform these exercises 3 days a week on alternate days. Here are some pointers for doing the following 11 exercises:

- Begin with a hand-held weight no heavier than 6 pounds (about 3 kilograms), then gradually progress to a maximum weight of 13 pounds (about 6 kilograms) or more if you can tolerate it.
- Do 8-16 complete and continuous executions (repetitions) for each exercise.
- Perform all these exercises 1 or more times, resting for between 15 and 60 seconds between sets—longer if necessary. Once you are able to perform two complete sets (2 × 16 repetitions for each exercise) with relative ease, you may want to switch to a heavier weight. However, keep in mind that it's more important to do the exercise correctly than to increase the amount of weight.
- Do not hold your breath during these repetitions. If you feel inclined to do so, the weight may be too heavy, causing you to strain too much.
- Maintain good posture throughout each exercise set.

Side Shoulder Raise (outer portion of the shoulder). Start with your arms hanging in front of your thighs, elbows slightly bent, and palms facing each other. Raise both dumbbells outwards to shoulder height simultaneously, keeping elbows slightly bent. Lower dumbbells to starting position and repeat.

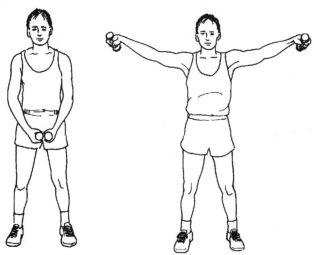

Figure 3.6

Front Shoulder Raise (front portion of the shoulder).   Begin with your arms hanging in front of your thighs and your palms facing the thighs. Raise one dumbbell straight in front of you to shoulder height. Lower this dumbbell to your starting position and repeat using other arm. Keep alternating your arms.

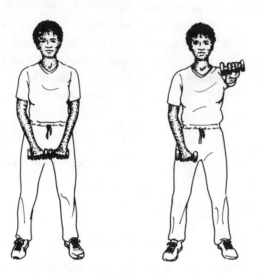

Figure 3.7

Bent-Over Shoulder Raise (rear portion of the shoulder and upper back).   Bend over until your torso is roughly parallel to floor. Keep your knees slightly bent. Start with your arms hanging down towards floor, palms facing inwards, and elbows slightly bent. Raise both dumbbells outward to shoulder height simultaneously, keeping elbows slightly bent. Lower dumbbells to starting position and repeat.

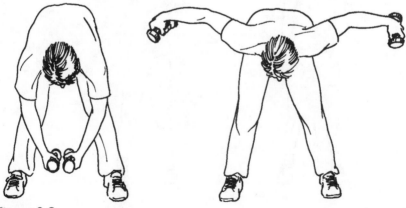

Figure 3.8

Upright Row (shoulder, neck, and upper back).   Stand with arms hanging in front of your thighs, palms facing your thighs, and the dumbbells close together. Keeping the palms close to the body, raise the dumbbells to the chin simultaneously. Lower the dumbbells to starting position and repeat.

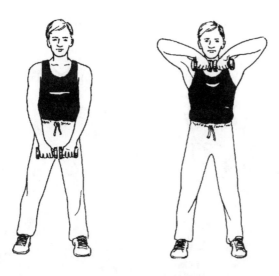

Figure 3.9

Bicep Curl (bicep, or front of the upper arm).   Start the exercise with your arms hanging at your sides and your palms facing in front of you. Keeping the elbows close to the sides of the body, curl both dumbbells upward to the shoulders. Lower and repeat.

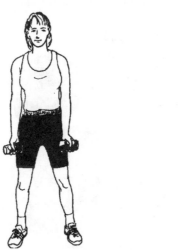
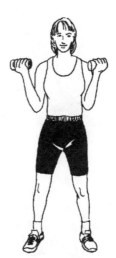

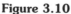

Figure 3.10

Tricep Extension (tricep, or back of the upper arm).   Place one foot about a step in front of the other and bend both knees slightly. Lean forward and rest one hand, palm down, on the knee of your front leg. Place the hand with the dumbbell in it against your hip (palm of your hand facing the hip). Keeping your elbow still, straighten your arm fully. Then bend your arm until your hand returns to your hip and repeat. After completing the desired number of repetitions, repeat with the other arm.

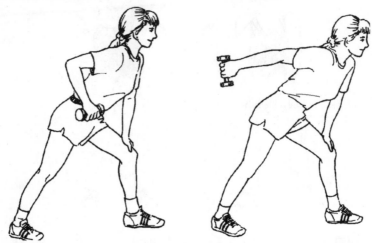

Figure 3.11

Supine Fly (chest muscles).   Lie face up on the floor with your knees bent and arms perpendicular to your body. Raise both dumbbells above your chest until they meet in the center. Lower dumbbells and repeat.

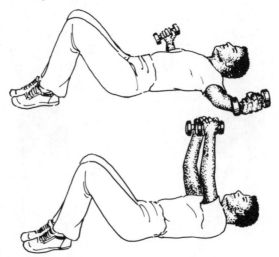

Figure 3.12

Pullover (chest and back). Lie face up on the floor. Begin with dumbbells together directly above the center of your chest, elbows slightly bent. Lower the dumbbells to the floor behind your head, keeping your elbows bent. Raise the dumbbells back to the starting position and repeat.

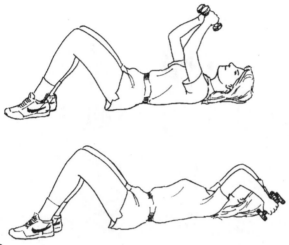

Figure 3.13

Sit-Ups (abdominal muscles). From a horizontal position, knees bent at a 90° angle and palms resting on your thighs, lift your shoulders off the ground and slide your fingers up toward your knees. Return to the starting position and repeat.

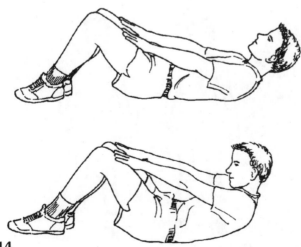

Figure 3.14

Calf Raises (calf muscles).   Start with your arms hanging at your sides, dumbbells in hand, and feet slightly apart. Raise up onto the balls of both feet. Lower your heels to the ground and repeat. Do not bend your knees.

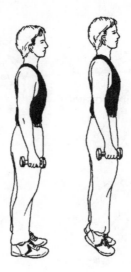

Figure 3.15

Lunges (thigh muscles and buttocks).   Start with your arms hanging at your sides, dumbbells in hands, and feet apart. Take one step forward with one foot and bend your front knee slightly. Step back to the starting position and repeat with the opposite leg. Keep alternating your legs.

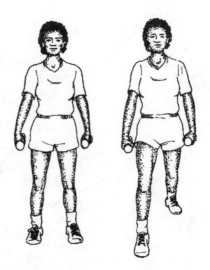

Figure 3.16

Isometric Muscle-Strengthening Exercises Using Resistance Rubber Bands

If your functional capacity has been severely impaired by CFS (see box on page 18 in chapter 2), you may find even my relatively easy muscle-strengthening program too strenuous. If so, you have two options. Research has shown that people like you can increase their strength substantially by following a strength-building program such as the one in the previous section but *without the weights.*[4] In effect, you'll be exercising against gravity.

Studies have also documented the fact that isometric exercises, which comprise my second program, can result in dramatic strength gains even though you'll probably find them far less strenuous. Isometric exercises are aimed at the skeletal muscles and involve the tensing of one set of muscles against another or against an immovable object such as a resistive rubber band. Such an exercise may involve placing the palms of your hands together and pushing, or gripping the sides of the chair you are sitting in and pulling up, holding the position for several seconds and then relaxing. Note that isometric exercises involve minimal or no joint movement.

If you find my first program too taxing, I urge you to spend 4 weeks or so doing these isometric exercises, then to gradually move into my regular muscle-strengthening program. Also, on days when your CFS flares up, and you feel too fatigued to do your regular workout, at least do some mild stretching and isometrics.

With one exception, all the exercises shown in Figures 3.17 to 3.21 use resistive rubber bands, which are relatively inexpensive (around $10 per band), versatile, and convenient to use. Different types are available. Dyna-Bands and Therabands, two of the most popular, can be ordered from The Hygenic Corporation, 1245 Home Ave., Akron, OH 44310, telephone 216-633-8460.

To exercise with them, you either pull or push against the bands, which resist your efforts. The amount of resistance varies according to the thickness of the band you're exercising with. The bands are color-coded to indicate their thickness and resistance. To do my isometric exercises, use the band that provides the most resistance and affords the least joint movement.

Here are specific pointers for doing the following five isometric exercises:

- Do 1-3 repetitions of each exercise daily.
- For these activities, tie your band to form a loop using a half-bow or a knot that is easy to undo.
- During the exercise, always try to maintain the natural width of the band. Don't let it fold over.
- During each repetition, push or pull as hard as you can for 6 seconds but never longer. Rest for 15-20 seconds between repetitions—longer if necessary. Between exercises, rest for 15-60 seconds.

Shoulder Press (shoulder and, to a lesser degree, the upper back). Place a looped band around your forearms, just above your wrists. Stand with your arms hanging in front of you, elbows slightly bent, and palms facing each other. Keeping your elbows slightly bent, try to push your arms outward as hard as possible and maintain the effort for 6 seconds. The band resistance should prevent your arms from moving more than a few inches if at all. Relax and either repeat or go on to the next exercise.

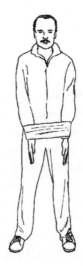

Figure 3.17

Chest Press (chest muscles and, to some extent, the upper back).
No bands are required for this exercise. Clasp your hands and extend
your arms out in front of you at chest height. Keeping your elbows
slightly bent, press the palms of your hands against each other as hard
as you can and maintain the effort for 6 seconds. Relax and either
repeat or go to the next exercise.

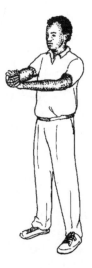

Figure 3.18

Combined Biceps Curl and Triceps Extension (biceps and the triceps).
Biceps are the muscles in the front of the upper arm; triceps are those
in the back of the upper arm. To strengthen them, place a looped
band around your forearms, just above your wrists. Hold both arms
gently against the front of your upper body, with your elbows bent at
about a 90° angle and one forearm just above the other. Turn the
palm of the top hand so that it's facing upwards and the palm of the
bottom hand so that it's facing downwards. For 6 seconds, try as hard
as you can to bend your top elbow and straighten your bottom elbow,
all the while keeping your forearms against your body. The resistance

of the band should keep elbow movement to a minimum. Relax and repeat the exercise, switching arm positions.

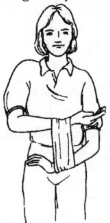

Figure 3.19

Standing Hip Flexion (hips, front of the thighs, and, to a lesser degree, abdominal muscles).   Stand between the backrests of two chairs with your feet close together. Place a looped band around the outsides of your ankles. Throughout this exercise, hold on to both backrests for balance and support, and keep both knees slightly bent. Bracing yourself with your arms and keeping one foot in place, press the other leg forward as hard as possible. The band's resistance should keep your leg from moving more than a few inches forward if at all. Maintain this stance for 6 seconds. Return your leg to the starting position and repeat with the opposite leg.

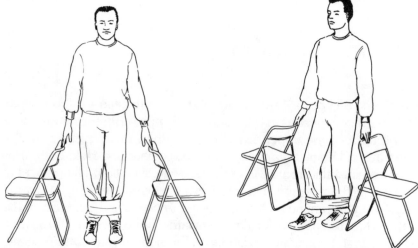

Figure 3.20

Standing Hip Extension (hips, back of the thighs, buttocks, and lower back muscles). This is a variation of Figure 3.20. Once again, you stand between two chairs with a looped band around the outsides of your ankles, holding on to the backrests of both chairs for balance and support, and keeping your knees slightly bent. Bracing yourself with your arms and keeping one foot in place, try to press the other leg backward as hard as possible. The band's resistance should prevent you from moving your leg more than a few inches backward if at all. Maintain this stance for 6 seconds. Return your leg to its starting position and repeat with the opposite leg.

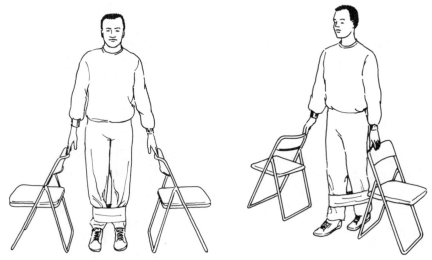

Figure 3.21

Performing Strength-Building Exercises Safely

Here are some pointers for doing all strength-building exercises correctly:

- Before you begin to exercise with rubber bands, remove all jewelry, even a watch, from your arms.
- Do not perform a Valsalva maneuver—that is, exhaling forcefully without releasing the air from the lungs—during lifting, pulling, or pushing. In short, *avoid holding your breath* because it increases stress on your cardiovascular system. If you feel inclined to do so, it could be a sign that the weight you're using is too heavy for your current strength level, or if you're using rubber bands, that you're pulling or pushing too hard. You shouldn't

have to strain. You may find it helpful to count out loud to make sure you're breathing normally.

- Do not undertake activities in which you must hold weight above your head for more than a few seconds. Such movements also place an excessive load on your cardiovascular system.
- When in doubt, substitute lighter weights for heavier weights and do more repetitions. Do not use heavier weights for the sake of shortening your exercise time. Heavier weights increase your blood pressure more than lighter ones.
- Prolonged isometric exercise can elicit adverse cardiac responses in patients with cardiovascular problems. Such people should *never hold a contraction for more than 6 seconds.*
- Maintain good posture throughout the exercise sequence.
- Start slowly and progress gradually. If you're very weak to start with, it won't take much exercise to improve your strength.

Aerobic Exercise

Ken Cooper actually coined the term "aerobics" in 1968 when his first book, *Aerobics*, was published.[5] Indeed, if you'd looked up the word *aerobic* in the dictionary before 1968, you might have found it described as an adjective meaning "growing in air or in oxygen." It was commonly used to describe bacteria that need oxygen to live. However, Ken used the word *aerobics* as a noun to denote those forms of endurance exercises that require increased amounts of oxygen for prolonged periods. Proof of Ken's influence came in the 1986 edition of the *Oxford English Dictionary* where *aerobics* is defined as "a method of physical exercise for producing beneficial changes in the respiratory and circulatory systems by activities which require only a modest increase of oxygen intake and so can be maintained."

For people with CFS, the tricky issue is determining how much aerobic exercise is enough to insure health benefits without increasing their chances of injury or becoming so exhausted that they have to stay in bed for several days to recover.

Dr. Steven N. Blair, Director of Epidemiology at The Cooper Institute for Aerobics Research, and other researchers from prestigious medical institutions in the United States have tackled this issue in depth.[6-8] They reviewed the findings of many exercise research studies and were able to identify an ideal upper and lower limit of exercise. While future studies are needed to clarify the situation fully, there appears to be a just-right level of exercise. This is actually a modest amount, far less than the extremely strenuous workouts that exercise enthusiasts engage in as a matter of course. In the language of exercise physiologists,

> Exercise training that results in a weekly energy expenditure of between *10 and 20 calories per kilogram of body weight** is likely to bring about the major health benefits.[6,7] Twenty calories is the upper limit necessary from a health promotion standpoint—energy expenditures above this level do not appear to provide substantially more benefit.[6] The lower limit of 10 calories is necessary to insure effectiveness,[7] although lesser amounts are still likely to be of some benefit.[9]

Here are two examples: Lisa Blake weighed 134 pounds (61 kilograms) when she first arrived at The Cooper Aerobics Center. Therefore, she needed to gradually build up to an energy expenditure of between 610 (61 × 10) and 1220 (61 × 20) calories during exercise each week. In contrast, another CFS patient, Steve White, weighed 187 pounds (85 kilograms). Therefore, his target weekly energy expenditure during exercise was 850 (85 × 10) to 1700 (85 × 20) calories.

These conclusions form the mathematical basis of the Health Points System you will encounter in the next chapter. Our Health Points System transforms these energy expenditure recommendations into a practical, easy-to-follow method of assessing the effectiveness of your exercise program. So, if you're concerned about the complexity of calculating your weekly energy expenditure, you can stop worrying—our Health Points System will take care of this for you. Without it, most CFS patients would have no way of knowing how much exercise is needed to expend 10 to 20 calories per kilogram of body weight.

Factors That Determine Energy Expenditure

Weekly energy expended during exercise depends largely on four factors: the *type, frequency, intensity,* and *duration* of your exercise sessions. Your doctor should discuss these four major considerations in deciding on a safe and effective weekly exercise regimen. Keeping both your medical condition and personal preferences in mind, your doctor must help you

---

*1 kilogram = approximately 2.2 pounds. 1 calorie = approximately 4.2 kilojoules.

- choose a suitable aerobic exercise,
- decide on the number of times you should work out each week,
- determine the appropriate intensity at which to perform exercise, and
- establish how long each exercise session should last.

It's important for you to understand how the last three items intertwine. They're embodied in the concept of FIT, which is an acronym for **Frequency, Intensity,** and **Time.** *Frequency* refers to *how often* you exercise. *Intensity* refers to *how hard* you exert yourself. *Time* refers to each exercise session's *duration.* An equation showing their interrelationship would look like this:

$$\text{Frequency} + \text{Intensity} + \text{Time} = \text{Caloric Energy Expenditure}$$
$$= \text{Health Benefit}$$

If the right side of the equation—that is, caloric energy expenditure and health benefit—is to remain constant but you cut down on one or two elements on the left side of the equation, the third element on the left side must increase to make up the difference. For example, if you exercise at a low-to-moderate intensity 3 days a week, each exercise session may have to last a relatively long time if you're to get enough exercise to have a substantial impact on your health. So if you exercise at that intensity but for a shorter length of time each session, you must increase the number of times per week you exercise to achieve the desired weekly energy expenditure.

Here are my recommendations concerning each of these factors:

Frequency.   I recommend 3 to 5 days per week as the ideal exercise schedule, both for healthy people and for those with CFS. Less frequency of exercise is unlikely to produce significant health improvements; more predisposes you to musculoskeletal injuries. You should space your workouts throughout the week. For example, if you're a 3-day-a-week exerciser, rather than training on Monday, Tuesday, and Wednesday, schedule your workouts for Monday, Wednesday, and Friday.

Time or Duration.   The higher the intensity or frequency, the shorter the time needed to attain the desired weekly energy expenditure. For most CFS patients, the ideal workout is 30 to 45 minutes long—not including the 5 minutes each of warm-up and cool-down. Moderate-intensity aerobic exercise of longer duration is preferable to high-intensity exercise of shorter duration for these reasons: (a) It lessens the risk of training-related medical complications, (b) it is less likely to worsen your fatigue and other CFS symptoms, particularly during the initial weeks of your exercise program, and (c) the average person is more likely to enjoy more moderate workouts. Longer, moderate workouts are particularly important if weight loss is a goal because they promote fat loss while reducing the risk of musculoskeletal injuries.

Workouts involving 30 to 45 minutes of continuous aerobic exercise are what most of you should aim to gradually build up to. However, because of your CFS, you might want to consider a viable alternative documented in studies at Stanford University. This research shows that three 10-minute exercise sessions spread throughout the day may result in fitness gains similar to one 30-minute session.[10] This finding should be welcome news to all CFS patients who find that extended exercise sessions make them too tired.

Another possibility is *interval training*. This means doing a series of bouts of exercise, with short rest periods between bouts, rather than one long, endurance-oriented workout. Here's how this might work: Instead of cycling for 30 minutes without stopping, you'd divide the session into six mini-sessions. You'd cycle for 5 minutes, then either cycle at a very low intensity or rest completely for 1 minute before the next session in order to reduce temporarily any fatigue you

Fitness gains through intermittent exercise sessions

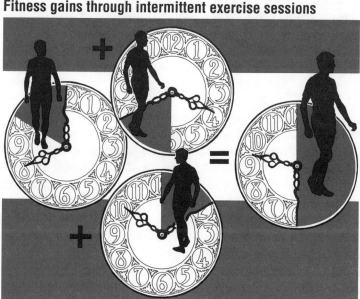

are experiencing. Incidentally, low-intensity exercise is preferable to a complete stop because abrupt cessation of exertion may cause a dangerous drop in your blood pressure.

Intensity.   It's a fallacy to assume that you must exercise at high intensities to derive health-related benefits. In short, the "no pain, no gain" axiom is wrong. It's an especially dangerous idea for people with CFS because it's likely to aggravate rather than alleviate fatigue and certain other CFS symptoms. Fortunately, it is now known that a person exercising at moderate rather than high intensity can derive optimal health-related benefits with a minimum of risk.

How to Quantify Exercise Intensity

There are a number of ways to quantify exercise intensity. I'll discuss three you can choose from: METs, your heart rate, or your perceived exertion.

METs.   The acronym MET stands for "metabolic equivalent unit." One MET is the amount of oxygen your body consumes for energy production each minute while you're at rest. If you're engaged in an activity corresponding to 5 METs, this means that your body is now taking up and using 5 times more oxygen than it did at rest. This is the amount your body now needs to fuel your working muscles, enabling them to produce the required amount of energy. (I'll return to the subject of METs later in this chapter when I discuss how to select an appropriate speed or work rate for the initial weeks of a walking or stationary cycling exercise program.)

Heart Rate.   This is perhaps the most widely used and helpful way to target exercise intensity. This method is based on the principle that there's a direct relationship between the increase in your body's oxygen uptake during exertion and the increase in your heart rate.

I advise patients with CFS to exercise at an intensity that raises the heart rate above 60% of their maximal heart rate but no higher than 85% (unless they're competitive athletes). That's an exercise training zone range spanning 25 percentage points. I have found that an exercise heart rate in the range of 60% to 75% of the maximal heart rate is ideal for most CFS patients.

What is "maximal heart rate"? It's the highest heart rate you are capable of attaining during exercise without becoming so fatigued you have to stop, or without developing significant cardiac abnormalities.

Maximal heart rate can differ considerably from one person to the next.

The most accurate way to determine your maximal heart rate is to take a treadmill or cycle exercise test. In medical jargon, this is called a "symptom-limited maximal exercise test with electrocardiogram (ECG) and blood pressure monitoring." (The term "symptom-limited" simply means that you continue exercising until you cannot go any further because you are too fatigued or you develop certain ECG or other abnormalities that are an indication for your physician to stop your test.) I strongly advocate this for all our CFS patients; I urge you to have one if at all possible.

Both Lisa Blake and Steve White had exercise tests. Lisa's maximal heart rate was 179 beats per minute. Steve's was 170 beats per minute. Without a test, you'll have to use one of the following formulas to *estimate* your maximal heart rate:

For all women and sedentary men:
220 minus your age in years = Estimated Maximal Heart Rate

For conditioned men:
205 minus one-half your age in years = Estimated Maximal Heart Rate

For example, Lisa Blake at age 34 had an estimated maximal heart rate of 186 beats per minute (220 − 34 = 186). At age 46, Steve White's estimated maximal heart rate was 174 beats per minute (220 − 46 = 174) before he embarked on our supervised exercise program; had he already been engaged in an exercise program at that time, it would have been 182 beats per minute (205 − 23 = 182). Note that Lisa's actual maximal heart rate was 179, slightly lower than her estimate. Steve's was also lower—170.

Be aware that these formulas are invalid for people taking beta-blockers or other medications that slow down the heart rate. For safety reasons, I also caution people who know they have heart disease to ignore these formulas whether they're taking medication or not. Heart patients *must* have an exercise test before starting an exercise program.

Almost all patients seen at the Cooper Clinic receive exercise tests. Over the years the Clinic has done more than 70,000 of these tests, the results of which form a useful data base for evaluating how various ailments affect people's aerobic capacity and endurance. Our own study of 101 Cooper Clinic patients with CFS and two other investigations done elsewhere show that, while most CFS patients' maximal heart rates are close to their age-predicted maximums estimated using the formulas given earlier, some have values that are much lower than expected.[11,12,13] Using this evidence, I've arrived at the following maximal heart rate guidelines, which are based on a CFS patient's degree of functional impairment (see box on page 18 in chapter 2):

- If you are a *minimally* or *moderately impaired* CFS patient, you should be able to use the formulas with reasonable assurance.
- If you're *severely impaired* by CFS, use the formulas but multiply the value you obtain by 0.95 to arrive at your maximal heart rate.
- If you're *debilitated* by CFS, use the formulas but multiply the value you obtain by 0.90 to arrive at your maximal heart rate.

Training Target Heart Rate Zone.   Once you know your maximal heart rate, it's easy enough to determine the parameters you should stay within when you exercise. I recommend that you push your heart rate above 60% of your maximal heart rate but go no higher than 75% (and definitely not above 85%). This is your *training target heart rate zone*, which you calculate by multiplying your maximal heart rate by the lower limit of 60% (or 0.6) and the upper limit of 75% (or 0.75).

Using Lisa's actual maximal heart rate of 179, she calculated a lower limit of 107 beats per minute (or $179 \times 0.6 = 107$) and an upper limit of 134 beats per minute ($179 \times 0.75 = 134$). Steve's training target heart rate zone was between 102 ($170 \times 0.6 = 102$) and 128 ($170 \times 0.75 = 128$) beats per minute.

This zone is important. Studies show that exercise performed at an intensity lower than 60% may net some health benefits but is unlikely to increase substantially your level of fitness.[14,15] Moreover, in lieu of exceeding the 60% mark, you'll probably have to lengthen your exercise session to well over an hour each time to attain the weekly health points total I recommend. On the other hand, if you're under time pressure and can only work out a maximum of 3 days a week or for short durations, you'll be forced to exercise near the upper limit of your training target heart rate zone to gain any appreciable health benefit.

Keep in mind that it's crucial never to exceed the 85% upper limit; the only exceptions are for competitive athletes. Why? Because during high-intensity exercise, certain metabolic changes take place in your working muscles, such as a build-up of lactic acid, that foster quick fatigue. Since you already suffer from premature fatigue, it makes no sense to bring it on even faster. Also, high-intensity exercise increases the chances of developing cardiac complications in susceptible people.

<u>Using Heart Rate to Guide Intensity.</u> For novice exercisers, the following questions and answers will help you use your heart rate as a guide to your exercise intensity:

- *How do I measure my heart rate during exercise?* The same way as at rest—by taking your pulse. (See Appendix B.)

- *How often during exercise should I calculate my heart rate?* Initially, you may need to check your heart rate as often as every 5 minutes. Once you are familiar with your own appropriate exercise intensity, though, you'll probably only need to do it a few times each workout. I generally recommend that you check your rate at the following times:

1. *Before starting to exercise.* If it is above 100 beats per minute and remains this high after 15 minutes or so of rest, don't exercise at all. Call your doctor and discuss your elevated rate.
2. *After you complete your warm-up.* If your heart rate is above your heart rate limit at this point, slow down until it drops below the limit. In this situation you performed your warm-up at too high an intensity. Start off slower next time.
3. *After you've been exercising at your peak intensity for about 5 minutes.* If it is above your limit, slow down and recheck it within 5 minutes.
4. *At the point when you stop the aerobic phase and begin your cool-down.*
5. *When you complete your cool-down.* If your heart rate isn't below 100 beats per minute, rest until it reaches this level. Only then take a shower or drive off in your car.

- *Can I rely on a portable heart rate monitor instead of checking my heart rate manually?* Commercially available meters generally are worn on the chest and provide continual monitoring of your heart rate by transmitting electrical signals to a special wristwatch or a computer that's also worn on your chest. You can usually program your heart rate limit into the device and it will set off an alarm if you exceed it. Provided you purchase a reliable model, such monitors can be a valuable aid, although they're certainly not a necessity. Consult a member of your health-care team before purchasing one. Ask him or her which type is more accurate. Then before you actually purchase a specific one, ask that team member to help you verify its accuracy while you're wearing it.

Perceived Exertion. One of the simplest ways to quantify your exercise intensity is to use the scale I've reproduced in Table 3.1. Named after its originator, the Swedish exercise physiologist Dr. Gunnar Borg who developed it in the early 1950s, the Borg scale helps you judge your exercise intensity based on your on-the-spot perception of how hard the exercise feels.[16] This "rating of perceived exertion" (or RPE) is outlined on a scale from 6 to 20, which you consult as you exercise or immediately afterwards. If you're exerting yourself at a level that you feel is fairly strenuous, you might assign your effort an RPE of 13. When you reach the all-out huffing-and-puffing stage, you would choose a much higher rating of about 17.

Table 3.1
Borg Perceived Exertion Scale

The original Borg system for rating physical exertion is based on an open-ended scale running from 6 (equal to exertion at rest) to 20 (extreme effort).

Rating of perceived exertion or RPE	Verbal description of RPE
6	
7	Very, very light
8	
9	Very light
10	
11	Fairly light
12	
13	Somewhat hard
14	
15	Hard
16	
17	Very hard
18	
19	Very, very hard
20	

Note. From G.A. Borg, "Psychophysical Bases of Perceived Exertion," *Medicine and Science in Sports and Exercise, 14,* pp. 377-387, 1982, © by The American College of Sports Medicine. Reprinted by permission.

In healthy exercisers and patients with mild CFS, an RPE of 12 to 13 should correspond to an exercise intensity of 60% to 75% of your maximal heart rate—your recommended training target heart rate zone. However, this may not be true for you if your CFS is more severe. It's my experience that many patients with moderate to severe CFS are less able than healthy exercisers to tolerate the fatiguing sensations of exertion.[17] The end result is that they report higher RPEs than other people. That's why RPEs of 14 to 15 more closely correspond to their training heart rate zone. In any event, unless you're a competitive athlete and your doctor has given the okay, I suggest that you never exceed a score of 15 during training—even if your heart rate is below your prescribed limit.

Ideally, you should use both your heart rate and RPE to monitor the intensity of your workouts. However, provided your doctor has assured you that you do not suffer from cardiovascular disease (such as coronary artery disease) you may rely entirely on your RPE, should you wish.

Basic Aerobic Exercises to Get You Started

No, aerobic exercises *don't* require excessive speed or strength but they *do* require that you place demands on your cardiovascular system. Examples are brisk walking, running, swimming, cross-country skiing, and cycling.

In contrast, "*anaerobic*" exercise, as the prefix implies, means "without oxygen." Sprinting is an anaerobic activity. It involves an all-out burst of effort and relies on metabolic processes that do not require oxygen for energy production. Such processes result in fatigue within a relatively short time.

Aerobic exercise is far better than anaerobic for people with CFS who want to improve their health, for these reasons: Energy expenditure is related to how much oxygen your working muscles use during exercise. Aerobic exercise obviously uses up more oxygen than anaerobic exercise. Also, because it's more moderate and you can do it longer without becoming excessively fatigued, aerobic exercise allows you to expend far more energy than anaerobic exercise. Furthermore, when you exercise aerobically, you can better monitor your heart rate and keep it within your prescribed limit. Anaerobic exercise is more likely to push your heart rate above that limit, which can be dangerous if you have cardiovascular disease.

The aerobic exercises I most commonly recommend for CFS patients who are beginning an exercise program are walking, stationary cycling, and, for those with only a minimal degree of functional impairment, jogging. Each has its advantages and disadvantages:

Basic aerobic exercises

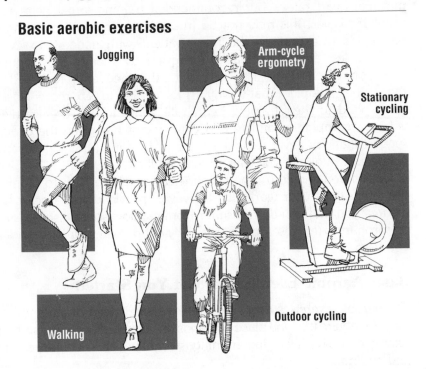

Jogging

Arm-cycle ergometry

Stationary cycling

Outdoor cycling

Walking

Walking.   Most experts, including me, consider walking one of the most appropriate aerobic activities for adults.[18] The intensity is easy to control, so even many CFS patients with moderate to severe functional impairment can walk and get the desired conditioning effect. It's simple and straightforward, requiring no special skill, setting, or equipment except a good pair of shoes. It is one of the least likely to cause musculoskeletal problems. And the findings of a recent study conducted by Drs. Tom R. Thomas and Ben R. Londeree suggest that at fast speeds the energy expenditure for walking approaches that for jogging.[19]

Jogging.   The advantages of jogging are similar to those for walking. The catch is that it generally requires greater exertion, or intensity, than walking, so it may often raise your heart rate and RPE above your designated limit. It may also increase your risk for musculoskeletal problems. However, if you're enthusiastic about jogging despite its greater risks, I recommend that you precede your jogging regimen with a walking program, then a walk-jog regimen.

Stationary Cycling. This is an activity busy people love. While you're pedaling away on your stationary cycle (also known as a *cycle ergometer*), you can do other things—read or watch TV, for example. Stationary cycling gives you no excuse should the weather make outdoor cycling impossible, and it causes less wear and tear on the musculoskeletal system than jogging.

Some stationary cycles, such as the Schwinn Air-Dyne, are a variation on the usual theme. They help you achieve higher energy expenditures by working your arms and legs simultaneously. You pump your legs up and down while you're moving your arms forward and back. The result is a more thorough upper- and lower-body workout. I recommend these cycle ergometers for many CFS patients, especially those who use their arms a lot in their work or recreation.

Outdoor Cycling. Outdoor cycling can be far more enjoyable and exhilarating than indoor cycling. The disadvantage over a stationary workout is that roads tend to go up and down. An unexpected incline could cause an excessive elevation in your heart rate or RPE. Also, too many downhill stretches and excessive delays in traffic and at stoplights may considerably lessen your energy expenditure and force you to increase the duration of your workouts in order to gain your desired energy expenditure. Then there is the danger that traffic poses. Still, if you can eliminate some of these drawbacks, outdoor cycling is great.

PUTTING ON THOSE WALKING SHOES AND VENTURING FORTH

Here are guidelines for beginning a walking, walk-jog, or stationary cycling exercise program. I recommend these forms of exercise to my sedentary adult CFS patients because they're a good way to slowly ease into the routine of regular exercise. After you've completed an introductory 8 weeks or so following one of the programs below, you'll be ready to start earning the 50 to 100 exercise health points I discuss in the next chapter.

Please note that these programs are only intended as a guideline. Your individual circumstances may require you to progress more slowly than suggested.

Beginning Walking Program

Walking is a wonderful way for CFS patients to get moving down the road to optimal health. But before you begin, you should ideally know your maximal MET value in order to estimate the speed (in mph or kph) at which you should walk during your first 8 weeks of exercise. Maximal MET value varies from one person to the next depending on his or her fitness level. If you've undergone an exercise test—which I urge all CFS patients to do—your doctor should be able to provide you with your maximal MET value. If not, err on the side of caution and start out at a comfortable speed that does not exceed what's recommended in Table 3.2 on page 60 for a person with a maximal MET value of 6. Regardless of whether or not you know your maximal MET value, I strongly advise against exceeding 75% of your maximal heart rate and an RPE of 13 during these initial weeks. Table 3.2 shows what your estimated beginning walking speed should be. Using this table, Lisa Blake, whose maximal MET value was 5, started her walking program at a speed of about 2.6 mph, or 4.2 kph.

The box on page 60 shows you what your walking program will look like in terms of each workout's duration and frequency.

Follow-Up Walk-Jog Program

Don't try jogging until you've followed a walking regimen for at least 6 weeks, ideally 12. You should be walking at a speed of at least 4 mph just before you graduate to jogging. If you're walking at a slower rate, you might as well stay with walking. Here are some pointers:

- When you start to jog, you should do so at a speed no faster than that at which you currently walk—and remember not to exceed the heart rate and RPE guidelines outlined earlier in this chapter.
- As always, warm up and cool down—each for at least 5 minutes. For the warm-up phase, walk briskly and try to raise gradually your heart rate to within at least 20 beats per minute of your target heart rate. Upon completing your jog, reduce gradually your speed to a slow walk over at least a 5-minute period.

The box on page 61 shows duration and frequency recommendations for your walk-jog program.

Beginning Stationary Cycling Program

If indoor cycling is more to your liking than walking, that's fine, for it's an excellent form of exercise.

Before you begin, you need to know your maximal MET value and your weight in pounds or kilograms (choose the weight closest to yours in Table 3.3). If you haven't had an exercise test and don't know your maximal MET value, start out at a comfortable work rate that does not exceed that recommended for a person with a maximal MET value of 7. Whether you know your maximal MET value or not, I strongly advise against exceeding 75% of your maximal heart rate and an RPE of 13 during these initial weeks. Table 3.3 on page 63 shows your estimated beginning work rate for a stationary cycling program. Steve White, who weighed 187 pounds (85 kg) and had a maximal MET value of 7, began his cycling program at 75 watts.

The duration and frequency recommendations for the first 8 weeks of your cycling program are shown in the box on page 63.

Beginning Schwinn Air-Dyne Cycling Program

A second form of indoor cycling, which works both your arms and legs, is the Schwinn Air-Dyne, another good choice for your early attempts to form a regular exercise habit. Table 3.4 shows how to estimate your work load for the first 8 weeks. If you don't know your maximal MET value, start at a comfortable work load of no more than what corresponds to a MET value of 7. Regardless of whether or not you know your maximal MET value, I strongly advise against exceeding 75% of your maximal heart rate and an RPE of 13 during these initial weeks. If you weigh 154 pounds (70 kg) and have a maximal MET value of 7, you would see by looking at Table 3.4 (page 64) that you should begin your Schwinn Air-Dyne cycling program at a work load of 1.3.

The box on page 64 shows duration and frequency recommendations for your Schwinn Air-Dyne program. Please be aware that there are a variety of other superb cycle ergometers that enable you to work your arms and legs simultaneously. Should you prefer to use one of them, these recommendations are equally applicable.

Beginning Program of Combined Walking and Stationary Cycling Using the Schwinn Air-Dyne

For people who get bored doing the same exercise day after day, I've devised an 8-week regimen that combines walking with cycling on the Schwinn Air-Dyne. This combination will also help reduce your risk of injury.

The guidelines for walking and Schwinn Air-Dyne workouts apply to this program. Estimate your starting walking speed and Schwinn

Air-Dyne work load for the first 8 weeks of this program using Tables 3.2 and 3.4.

You may start with either activity. As always, warm up for at least 5 minutes. After completing the first activity, proceed immediately to the other one—another warm-up is not needed. Upon completion of the second activity, cool down for at least 5 minutes.

The duration and frequency recommendations for your combined walking and Schwinn Air-Dyne program are shown in the box on page 65.

THAT ALL-IMPORTANT TRAINING LOG

I encourage all our CFS patients to keep track of their exercise efforts, at least in the beginning. A log provides you and your doctor with useful data. Moreover, it will help you be consistent with your exercise program. Following is an empty training log page. Make a number of photocopies and put them in a looseleaf notebook. Fill in a page after each day's worth of exercise.

DAILY EXERCISE TRAINING LOG

Date _____ Time of day _____ Body weight _____

Where I worked out _____

Resting pulse _____

Pre-exercise oral temperature (if measured) _____

Duration of stretching & muscle-strengthening _____

Pulse rate after stretching & muscle-strengthening

   (in beats per minute) _____

Aerobic portion of workout

   Type of exercise _____

   Duration (in minutes) _____

   Distance covered or work rate/load _____

   Highest heart rate _____

   Borg RPE (at most intense part of workout) _____

   Any symptoms experienced _____

Enjoyment rating   ____ 1 Very unenjoyable

               ____ 2 Unenjoyable

               ____ 3 Somewhat unenjoyable

               ____ 4 Enjoyable

               ____ 5 Very enjoyable

Health points earned (see chapter 4) _____

Table 3.2
Estimated Speed at Which to Begin a Walking Program

Maximal MET value	Estimated walking speed (miles per hour)	Estimated walking speed (kilometers per hour)
4	1.8 mph	2.9 kph
5	2.6 mph	4.2 kph
6	3.4 mph	5.4 kph
7 and above	4 mph	6.4 kph

Walking Program

Week	Duration per session	Frequency per week
1	10 minutes	3-5 times
2	15 minutes	3-5 times
3	20 minutes	3-5 times
4	25 minutes	3-5 times
5	30 minutes	3-5 times
6	35 minutes	3-5 times
7	40 minutes	3-5 times
8	45 minutes	3-5 times
9 and onward	It's time to start earning those 50 to 100 health points a week. Keep your exercise time at 45 minutes per session and gradually increase your speed until you exceed 60% of your maximal heart rate (if you are not doing so yet). If this does not result in the desired weekly energy expenditure using the health points charts in chapter 4,* do one or more of the following: Try exercising within the upper range of your target heart rate zone; exercise more frequently; or increase the duration of each exercise session.	

*At fast speeds, the energy you expend for walking approaches that for jogging. Therefore, for speeds of 4 mph (or 6.4 kph) or faster, I recommend that you use our jogging chart in chapter 4 to calculate your health points.

Walk-Jog Program		
Week	**Duration per session**	**Frequency per week**
1	*20 minutes total*—Walk 4.5 min, jog 0.5 min, walk 4.5 min, jog 0.5 min, walk 4.5 min, jog 0.5 min, walk 4.5 min, jog 0.5 min*	3-5 times
2	*20 minutes total*—Walk 4 min, jog 1 min, walk 4 min, jog 1 min, walk 4 min, jog 1 min, walk 4 min, jog 1 min*	3-5 times
3	*20 minutes total*—Walk 3 min, jog 2 min, walk 3 min, jog 2 min, walk 3 min, jog 2 min, walk 3 min, jog 2 min*	3-5 times
4	*20 minutes total*—Walk 2 min, jog 3 min, walk 2 min, jog 3 min, walk 2 min, jog 3 min, walk 2 min, jog 3 min*	3-5 times
5	*20 minutes total*—Walk 5 min, jog 5 min, walk 5 min, jog 5 min*	3-5 times
6	*20 minutes total*—Walk 4 min, jog 6 min, walk 4 min, jog 6 min*	3-5 times
7	*20 minutes total*—Walk 3 min, jog 7 min, walk 3 min, jog 7 min*	3-5 times
8	*20 minutes total*—Jog 10 min, walk 10 min*	3-5 times
9	*20 minutes total*—Jog 12 min, walk 8 min*	3-5 times

(Cont.)

Walk-Jog Program (Cont.)		
Week	Duration per session	Frequency per week
10	*20 minutes total*—Jog 15 min, walk 5 min*	3-5 times
11	*20 minutes total*—Jog 17 min, walk 3 min*	3-5 times
12	*20 minutes total*—Jog 20 min*	3-5 times
13 and onward	By the time you reach this point, you are likely to have exceeded 60% of your maximal heart rate; and you've possibly attained your desired weekly energy expenditure—100 health points per week —using the health points charts in chapter 4.* If so, just keep following week 12's regimen. If, on the other hand, you haven't been able to exceed 60% of your maximal heart rate, increase your speed. If that does not result in 100 weekly health points, do one or more of the following: Try exercising within the upper range of your target heart rate zone; exercise more frequently; or increase the duration of each exercise session.	

*You may find that you are below your desired weekly energy expenditure during the early weeks of this walk-jog effort. You can compensate by walking longer at the end of the jogging phase, before starting your cool-down. Use the jogging chart in chapter 4 when calculating your health points for your walk-jog program.

Table 3.3
Estimated Work Rate at Which to Begin a Stationary Cycling (Legs Only) Program

	Work rate (watts)					
Maximal MET value	Body weight = 110 lb (50 kg)	Body weight = 132 lb (60 kg)	Body weight = 154 lb (70 kg)	Body weight = 176 lb (80 kg)	Body weight = 198 lb (90 kg)	Body weight = 220 lb (100 kg)
4	20	25	29	33	37	41
5	29	35	41	47	53	58
6	38	46	53	61	68	76
7	47	56	65	75	84	93
8 and above	55	67	78	89	100	111

Stationary Cycling Program

Week	Duration per session	Frequency per week
1	7.5 minutes	3-5 times
2	10 minutes	3-5 times
3	12.5 minutes	3-5 times
4	15 minutes	3-5 times
5	17.5 minutes	3-5 times
6	20 minutes	3-5 times
7	25 minutes	3-5 times
8	30 minutes	3-5 times
9 and onward	It's time to start earning those 50 to 100 health points a week. Keep your exercise time at 30 minutes per session and gradually increase your work rate until you exceed 60% of your maximal heart rate (if you are not doing so yet). If this does not result in the desired weekly energy expenditure using the health points charts in chapter 4, do one or more of the following: Try exercising within the upper range of your target heart rate zone; exercise more frequently; or increase the duration of each exercise session.	

Table 3.4
**Estimated Work Load at Which to Begin
a Schwinn Air-Dyne Cycling Program**

	Work load					
Maximal MET value	Body weight = 110 lb (50 kg)	Body weight = 132 lb (60 kg)	Body weight = 154 lb (70 kg)	Body weight = 176 lb (80 kg)	Body weight = 198 lb (90 kg)	Body weight = 220 lb (100 kg)
4	.4	.5	.6	.7	.7	.8
5	.6	.7	.8	.9	1.1	1.2
6	.8	.9	1.1	1.2	1.4	1.5
7	.9	1.1	1.3	1.5	1.7	1.9
8 and above	1.1	1.3	1.6	1.8	2	2.2

Schwinn Air-Dyne Program		
Week	**Duration per session**	**Frequency per week**
1	7.5 minutes	3-5 times
2	10 minutes	3-5 times
3	12.5 minutes	3-5 times
4	15 minutes	3-5 times
5	17.5 minutes	3-5 times
6	20 minutes	3-5 times
7	25 minutes	3-5 times
8	30 minutes	3-5 times
9 and onward	It's time to start earning those 50 to 100 health points a week. Keep your exercise time at 30 minutes per session and gradually increase your work load until you exceed 60% of your maximal heart rate (if you are not doing so yet). If this does not result in the desired weekly energy expenditure using the health points charts in chapter 4, do one or more of the following: Try exercising within the upper range of your target heart rate zone; exercise more frequently; or increase the duration of each exercise session.	

Combined Walking and Schwinn Air-Dyne Program

Week	Duration per session		Frequency per week
	Walking	**Schwinn Air-Dyne**	
1	5 minutes	5 minutes	3-5 times
2	7.5 minutes	7.5 minutes	3-5 times
3	10 minutes	10 minutes	3-5 times
4	12.5 minutes	12.5 minutes	3-5 times
5	15 minutes	15 minutes	3-5 times
6	17.5 minutes	17.5 minutes	3-5 times
7	20 minutes	20 minutes	3-5 times
8	22.5 minutes	22.5 minutes	3-5 times

9 and onward   It's time to start earning those 50 to 100 health points a week. Keep the combined exercise time at 45 minutes per session and gradually increase the intensity until you exceed 60% of your maximal heart rate (if you're not doing so yet). If this does not result in the desired weekly energy expenditure using the health points charts in chapter 4, do one or more of the following: Try exercising within the upper range of your target heart rate zone; exercise more frequently; or increase the duration of each exercise session.

Chapter 3

Prescription

☐ Start your exercise program slowly and progress gradually, as your condition permits.

☐ Always include both a warm-up and a cool-down of at least 5 minutes' duration in each of your exercise sessions.

☐ Do stretching and, unless contraindicated, aerobic exercises 3 to 5 times each week.

☐ Include muscle-strengthening exercises in your exercise routines 2 to 3 times each week.

☐ If your functional capacity has been severely impaired by CFS, make use of isometric muscle-strengthening exercises for at least 4 weeks before progressing to a more strenuous strength-building program.

☐ Use isometric muscle-strengthening exercises when your CFS flares up and you feel too fatigued to do your regular workout.

☐ Structure the aerobic portion of your workout so that it is eventually 15 to 60 minutes long.

☐ Aim for an exercise intensity that raises your heart rate to between 60% and 75% of your maximal value and elicits an RPE of 12 to 13 during the aerobic portion of your workout.

☐ Don't exceed 85% of your maximal heart rate or an RPE of 15 at any point in your workout.

☐ Make use of interval training to lessen your fatigue during exercise.

☐ When your CFS flares up de-intensify your workouts.

☐ Exercise your options: Choose aerobic exercises that are convenient to perform.

☐ Keep track of your exercise efforts in a training diary.

Chapter 4

The Health Points System: Insuring Maximum Health Benefits With Minimum Risk

In trying to motivate CFS patients to follow exercise prescriptions, I always feel I'm walking several fine lines. First, as a physician, I have to educate patients adequately so their excuse can never be "I didn't understand." Then I must alert them to the seriousness of their condition and the risks involved in exercise without making them feel it's hopeless. I also need to emphasize the benefits of regular, moderate exercise, which can spell the difference between health and disability. Most importantly, I have to impress on patients the fact that drugs and medical care can go only so far in making them well. They must do the rest by making positive lifestyle changes, including exercise. With our Health Points System, you can chart how effective your exercise program is likely to be in promoting your health.*

In all aspects of life, we humans like to get report cards that let us know where we stand in our various endeavors. Our Health Points System is a kind of report card on your exercise program, except that you fill it out, not a doctor or a teacher. Our Health Points System enables you to quantify one constructive lifestyle change you can easily undertake to improve your health and reduce your chronic fatigue and certain other CFS symptoms. It allows you to chart your progress mathematically so you can see, in black and white, what you are accomplishing with exercise and where you stand.

We devised our Health Points System so that patients would do just enough exercise to gain optimal health benefits without exerting themselves to the point at which exercise becomes risky. Our system incorporates the two goals of effectiveness and safety. As a person with CFS, you must strike a fine balance between the two.

HOW THE HEALTH POINTS SYSTEM WORKS

As I explained in chapter 3, our system is based on the number of calories people of various weights expend during exercise. From my and other doctors' and exercise physiologists' experience and studies, it is known that

> aerobic exercise performed for 15 to 60 minutes per workout 3 to 5 days each week at an intensity that raises the heart rate to between 60% and 85% of the maximal value will result in an energy expenditure that brings about the desired health benefits.

If you're a novice exerciser, you should follow one of the beginning exercise programs I outlined in chapter 3 to work your body up gradually to an appropriate level of exertion. Although you can start using the Weekly Health Points Exercise Tally Sheet (see page 69) during this time, you should not try specifically to earn 50 to 100 health points until at least week 9. Depending on the severity of your CFS, it may take you far longer than this to earn the desired number of points. That's fine. It's the regularity of your exercise effort that counts the most in the beginning. Be patient.

---

*Those of you with relatively mild CFS and no other chronic diseases have the option of following Ken Cooper's well-known Aerobic Point System instead of our Health Points System. He describes it fully in *The Aerobics Program for Total Well-Being*.[1]

WEEKLY HEALTH POINTS EXERCISE TALLY SHEET

Your Weekly Goal: To earn between 50 and 100 health points each week, which corresponds to an expenditure of 10 to 20 calories per kilogram (2.2 pounds) of body weight per week. Exceeding this upper limit does not provide substantially more health benefit; thus you should keep your weekly health points total at, or very near, 100. To gain optimal benefit, you should earn your weekly quota of points across at least 3 workouts.

To find out how many health points you earned during an exercise session, simply use the chart (see Tables 4.1-4.5, pages 81-88) that corresponds to the form of aerobic exercise you're doing and fill in the results below:

Monday	Tuesday	Wednesday	Thursday	Friday	Saturday	Sunday		Total weekly health points
____ pt. +	____ pt. +	____ pt. +	____ pt. +	____ pt. +	____ pt. +	____ pt.	=	____ pt. (100 pt. maximum)

INTERPRETING THE EFFECTIVENESS OF YOUR WEEKLY EXERCISE EFFORT*

100 health points from exercise	Ideal. *You couldn't do better!*
70-99 health points from exercise	Very good. *Be proud of yourself.*
50-69 health points from exercise	Good. *But you could do better.*
20-49 health points from exercise	Fair. *Try a bit harder.*
10-19 health points from exercise	Poor. *But it's better than nothing.*
Less than 10 health points from exercise	Very poor. *Come on, now.*

*If your CFS or other medical conditions are such that you cannot attain the desired weekly number of health points, ignore this interpretation. Be proud of whatever progress you are able to make.

Precisely how many weekly health points should you aim for, 50 or 100? The answer depends on your current degree of functional impairment (see box on page 18 in chapter 2). If you're *minimally impaired*, aim for the full quota of 100 health points. If you're *moderately impaired*, aim for between 70 and 100 health points. If you're *severely impaired*, aim for between 50 and 70 health points. And if you're *debilitated* by CFS, try gradually to work your way up to 50 health points if possible.

You should follow our health points program for the rest of your life in order to remain at as optimal a state of well-being as possible. However, I'm aware that if you are incapacitated or in an invalid state because of CFS, you may not be able to attain the desired weekly number of health points. Even if you aren't incapacitated, you may not earn the desired number of points because you decide to do an exercise for which I don't provide a points chart. Don't brood over any of these roadblocks. Provided you perform some type of aerobic exercise for a minimum of 15 minutes at least 3 days a week, you'll get important health-related benefits, to be sure. Rather than attempt to fulfill expectations that may be unrealistic given your present clinical circumstances, be proud of whatever progress you can make. Also keep in mind when referring to our interpretation of the effectiveness of your weekly exercise effort on the tally sheet, that *it is not applicable to persons whose medical condition (as opposed to factors such as a lack of interest or desire) prevents them from attaining the recommended weekly number of health points.*

HOW TO USE OUR HEALTH POINTS CHARTS

The only way people can get a truly accurate fix on their energy expenditure during exercise is through laboratory testing. Technicians can use sophisticated equipment to measure the exact amount of oxygen the body takes up during a workout. The charts that follow are derived from numerous exercise research studies performed in such laboratories.

The health points charts found at the end of this chapter (Tables 4.1-4.4) cover walking, jogging, stationary cycling, and the Schwinn Air-Dyne—all forms of exercise described in depth in chapter 3. It was possible to formulate charts for these forms of exercise because (a) none require much skill, and (b) there's a great deal of outstanding research data available for them.

If you're exercising on equipment that I have not provided charts for but which gives you a readout of the number of calories you've expended, you can also easily convert such a number to health points. Divide the read-out number (calories) by the number you get when you divide your body weight (in pounds) by 11. If your body weight is in kilograms, divide the read-out number by the number you get when you divide your kilogram weight by 5. For example, if the read-out number is 120 calories and you weigh 165 pounds (75 kilograms), you've earned 8 health points (165 pounds ÷ 11, or 75 kilograms ÷ 5, = 15 and 120 calories ÷ 15 = 8 health points).

To determine the health points you earn for walking and jogging, you need to know the distance you covered during your workout, and the time it took you. If you're lucky enough to have access to a measured running track, figuring the distance will pose no problem. Otherwise you might want to invest in a pedometer or use your car's odometer to stake out a stretch of road to use as a track. You'll need a watch with a second hand or a stopwatch to measure accurately the duration of your exercise session.

To ascertain your health points on the charts for stationary cycling and the Schwinn Air-Dyne, you'll need to know the duration of your workout, your work rate (wattage) or work load (for the Schwinn Air-Dyne), and your weight.

To show you how easy the Health Points System is to use, on pages 72 and 73 are some examples from Lisa Blake's training diary, which show the number of health points she earned for each activity. At the time of "Week A," which was 12 weeks into her training program, Lisa weighed 130 pounds (about 59 kilograms). During "Week B," some 6 months later, her weight was down to 121 pounds (55 kilograms) due to her improved eating and exercising habits. This schedule enabled Lisa to earn our optimal weekly recommended goal of 100 health points.

OTHER AEROBIC EXERCISE CHOICES: THE PROS AND CONS

Table 4.5, also at the end of the chapter, is a chart labeled "Other Aerobic Activities." In order to vary your routine, you may want to try some of these other forms of exercise. When doing so, keep in

Week A

Date	Activity	Time	Distance/ work load	Health points	Notes
S					
M	Walk	22-1/2 min	1-1/4 miles	7.6	*12 weeks ago I wouldn't have*
	Schwinn Air-Dyne	22-1/2 min	1.0 WL	10.8	*believed I could walk this far!*
T					
W	Walk	20 min	1-1/10 miles	6.5	*Tired today but felt good*
	Cycle (legs)	20 min	55 watts	10	*after workout.*
T					
F	Walk	15 min	8/10 mile	4.9	*Felt good today.*
	Schwinn Air-Dyne	25 min	1.0 WL	12	
S					
				51.8	**Total: Week 12**

mind that these other forms of aerobic exercise either require skill, are influenced by external factors such as the weather or terrain, or have not been intensively researched. Thus, although this table is extremely useful, it isn't quite as precise as those for walking, jogging, and stationary cycling. To use this table you need to know how long you exercised and whether you exercised at a light (RPE < 12), moderate (RPE = 12-13), or high (RPE > 13) intensity.

Week B

Date	Activity	Time	Distance/ work load	Health points	Notes
S	Walk	45 min	3-1/2 miles	35.9	Tough day. I didn't think I'd finish.
M					
T	Aerobics class	30 min	12 RPE	15.9	I really enjoy this class!
W					
T	Aerobics class	30 min	12 RPE	15.9	Good workout.
F					
S	Walk	45 min	3-1/2 miles	35.9	Walked with Theresa today & didn't notice much exertion.
				103.6	**Total: Week 36**

The ideal aerobic exercise for you has three basic characteristics:

- It's pleasant. An exercise you enjoy is one you're more likely to stick with.
- It is practical and fits into your lifestyle—something you can perform conveniently all year round.

• It uses large muscle groups. Why is this important? Because the larger the muscle groups involved in your exercise effort, the greater your body's oxygen uptake and, hence, energy expenditure. In addition to the exercises already discussed, all of the following exercises, and many others, fulfill this criterion.

Swimming

This is an excellent aerobic activity because it incorporates both the upper and the lower body musculature. And because it's a nonweight-bearing activity, the risk of musculoskeletal injury is extremely low. I find swimming especially valuable for people with lower back problems, arthritis, or heat-regulation disorders.

If you're overweight, one of your exercise goals should be to shed pounds. Unfortunately, recent research indicates that swimming may not help you as much in this regard as some other forms of aerobic exercise.[2] Although the precise reason for this is not known, it may be because swimming causes the body temperature to rise less than other aerobic activities. Further research is needed to clarify this issue.

Aqua-Aerobics

This is just what the name implies: aerobic exercises done in water. The advantages and disadvantages of this increasingly popular low-impact sport are similar to those for swimming. If you find the prospect of exercising in a swimming pool appealing, consult Ken Cooper's book, *Overcoming Hypertension*, for detailed guidelines.[3]

Cross-Country Skiing

Ken Cooper rates this as the top aerobic activity. Ken's reasoning: "You have more muscles involved than just the legs; and any time you get more muscles involved, you get more aerobic benefit."[4] The heavy clothing you wear and the weighty equipment you must carry further enhance the aerobic effect (that is, your energy expenditure) over that of walking or jogging at similar speeds.

There are drawbacks. The total exertion is greatly affected by variations in skill, snow surface, terrain, temperature and weather conditions, and altitude. Also, it's difficult to take your pulse in the middle of this activity. And, some CFS patients find that cold weather aggravates their symptoms. One way around these barriers is mechanical cross-country skiing devices, which some of our patients enjoy using. These devices not only enable you to burn off calories efficiently, but because the activity is low-impact, they are unlikely to cause musculoskeletal problems.

Stair Climbing

A testament to the current popularity of stair-climbing machines is that they always seem to be in use at health clubs. These machines let you simulate the act of climbing flights of stairs, thus allowing you to work the large muscles in your back, buttocks, and legs and expend large amounts of energy in a relatively short time. Because stair climbing is strenuous, it's generally not a good way for beginners—especially those with CFS—to start exercising. If the idea of stair climbing appeals to you, wait until you've been working out for at least 8 weeks, before incorporating it into your exercise regimen.[5]

People with knee problems may need to find another way to get an aerobic workout, because the stress stair climbing places on the knee joint is thought to be equivalent to lifting four to six times your body weight. Needless to say, it's likely to aggravate existing problems in that area.[5]

Rope Skipping

This is a practical, enjoyable, and easily accessible aerobic activity. However, it's not a popular choice because it's relatively strenuous and may result in excessively high heart rates. It has the disadvantage of raising the heart rate with less energy expenditure than some other strenuous aerobic exercises such as jogging. Moreover, it exposes you to the risk of musculoskeletal disorders, a significant drawback.

Rebounding

Rebounding means running in place on a minitrampoline. Its advantage is that it reduces the risk of overexertion and injury. Its main disadvantage is that it limits your energy expenditure. The trampoline does too much of the work, causing your legs to spring up with little exertion on your part. Therefore, rebounding may be a suitable activity during the very early phase of your exercise program, but it may have to be abandoned in favor of a more vigorous exercise later on.[6]

Aerobic Dance

Aerobic dancing is steady, rhythmic movement done to the beat of relatively fast music. Recently benches ranging in height from 6 to 12 inches (15 to 30 centimeters) have been introduced into aerobic dance workouts to increase the exercise intensity and reduce the impact and risk of injury.[7] While there's no denying that many people adore aerobic dance, bench aerobics and even many traditional aerobics classes are often too strenuous for CFS patients. If you do choose this form of exercise, you must be vigilant about working at your own pace and staying within your heart rate and RPE limits.

Circuit Resistance Training

This is a combination of aerobics and strength training. Typically an exerciser would use a series of strength training machines and move from one to another with very short rest periods in between (usually 15 to 30 seconds). Circuit training has been touted as a way to improve the cardiovascular system, build and tone muscles, and burn calories during one carefully constructed workout.

Sounds great, doesn't it?

I didn't want to dismiss this exercise option out of hand so I reviewed the medical literature and did my own study of its possible rehabilitation benefits.[8] Here's the catch: The primary benefit is enhancement of muscular strength, not improvement in aerobic fitness and the cardiovascular system. Thus, I do not recommend it for anyone with CFS unless it's performed in conjunction with other forms of aerobic exercise. Even then, I think many of you may find it too strenuous during the early weeks of your training program.

Recreational Sports

People with relatively mild CFS and no other chronic diseases can participate in just about any exercise and sport. Likewise, people with more severe CFS and those with other chronic diseases are often able to take part in recreational sports, provided they stay within their heart rate and RPE limits. To do this, you may have to modify the rules of a game somewhat. When performed this way, recreational sports can be a valuable component of a CFS rehabilitation exercise program.

A word of caution about contact sports, such as football: CFS can involve your lymph system; either you or your doctor will be able to detect lymph nodes that are painful or enlarged. If your spleen, your body's largest lymph gland, is enlarged, it will be more susceptible to injury during rough sports. Therefore, it's a good idea for CFS patients to check with their doctor before participating in such activities.

Although I have not included sample introductory programs for each of these alternative exercise choices, you should be able to use the walking and stationary cycling programs at the end of chapter 3 as prototypes for your own programs. For example, an introductory swimming program might be as follows:

Week	Duration per session	Frequency per week
1	7.5 minutes	3-5 times
2	10 minutes	3-5 times
3	12.5 minutes	3-5 times
4	15 minutes	3-5 times
5	17.5 minutes	3-5 times
6	20 minutes	3-5 times
7	25 minutes	3-5 times
8	30 minutes	3-5 times
9 and onward	It's time to start earning those 50 to 100 health points a week. Keep your exercise time at 30 minutes per session and gradually increase your swimming speed until you exceed 60% of your maximal heart rate (if you are not doing so yet). If this does not result in the desired weekly energy expenditure using the Other Aerobic Activities chart (Table 4.5, page 86), do one or more of the following: Try exercising within the upper range of your target heart rate zone; exercise more frequently; or increase the duration of each exercise session.	

In using this swimming program, as with any aerobic exercise, begin at a comfortable intensity. During the initial weeks you would not exceed 75% of your maximal heart rate and an RPE of 13. You would also be sure to warm up and cool down—each for at least 5 minutes. This could be done with the use of slower swimming or other activities in the water.

Other aerobic choices

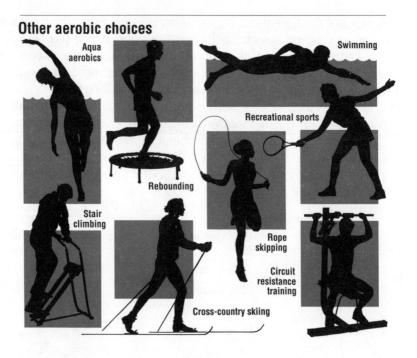

Aqua aerobics

Swimming

Recreational sports

Rebounding

Stair climbing

Rope skipping

Circuit resistance training

Cross-country skiing

THE FOUR-LETTER WORD
YOU MUST NOT UTTER

That word is "quit."

You've probably noticed I keep pushing the notion of *regular* exercise—not sporadic exercise, not fair-weather exercise, but the kind of persistent exercise you engage in almost daily because it's a habit, like brushing your teeth. There's a reason. When you exercise, your body and its various organ systems are being exposed to potent physiologic stimuli. If you exercise on a regular basis at an appropriate intensity and duration, these stimuli result in specific adaptions your body makes that both enhance your ability to exercise and, at the same time, improve your health status. In other words, you'll be the happy recipient of all the benefits of a physically active lifestyle, benefits outlined in chapter 2.

Unfortunately, these benefits can't be stored up for a rainy day. They're reversible. All it takes to set this backtracking in motion is abstinence. If you stop training or reduce your level of physical activity below your required level, your body's systems soon readjust themselves to this diminished amount of physiologic stimuli. The end result: Those hard-won, exercise-related gains, which you worked so long and hard to achieve, are lost.

This "reversibility concept" is shown best in a landmark study of some 16,936 Harvard University alumni by Dr. Ralph S. Paffenbarger, Jr. and his colleagues.[9] In this study, many former college athletes became inactive adults. As a consequence, they were in worse shape—and at greater risk for cardiovascular disease—than their contemporaries who had not participated in sports in college but who started exercising later in life. Researchers do not know how long it takes after you stop training before all the health benefits of exercise are lost. We do know that even after many months of training, a rapid decline in fitness occurs during the first 12 to 21 days of inactivity, and the fitness benefits of regular exercise are almost totally lost after about 2 or 3 months.[10]

In view of this, it's imperative that you stick with your exercise program once you get started. This is easier said than done. A number of studies focusing on exercise compliance show that half or more of all patients drop out of their exercise program within 6 months. The critical drop-out period for CFS patients is probably the initial 8 weeks or so because exercise may tend to make them feel somewhat worse during this fragile transition period, when their body is still becoming reaccustomed to exertion. You need motivators to get you through this critical time. The following suggestions will keep you huffing and puffing even when you'd rather be home in bed or watching television:

• *Make sure you fully understand the costs of not exercising versus the benefits of exercising.*

• *Start exercising slowly and progress gradually.* If you follow the beginning programs outlined in this book, this is just what you'll be doing.

• *Choose a form of exercise that's convenient as well as enjoyable.* Should you constantly score below a "4" on the enjoyment rating checklist in the exercise log on page 59, your exercise program needs to be modified in some way.

• *Find a role model*—a friend, relative, or acquaintance who leads a physically active life. Find out why they love exercise so much.

• *Learn from your past exercise experiences.* Try to determine where you went wrong previously.

• *Obtain as much support for your exercise program as possible.* Enlist the company, or at the very least the moral support, of those closest to you. On the other hand, you must never let peer pressure force you to exercise more strenuously than you should. Although exercising with others has many advantages, always work at your own pace. You've got a special condition—CFS—and even if your exercise companion has it too, their case won't necessarily be the same as yours. While goals are important as exercise motivators, I urge you to keep yours realistic and modify them continually as your condition changes.

• *Bring your body to your place of exercise, even if your mind is temporarily on strike.* Often it's just a matter of overcoming mental inertia. A body at rest prefers to remain at rest. But once you start exercising, you may find you enjoy it more than you anticipated. Remember, special occasions, such as holidays or vacations, are no excuse.

• *Finally, remember that exercise lasts a lifetime.* A diamond may be forever, they say in the beautiful, full-color advertisements for engagement rings. The same can be said about exercise, for physical activity is a lifelong pursuit.

I exhort you to do everything in your power to keep from becoming an exercise dropout, especially during the crucial initial months. Once you've passed the 6-month mark and tasted some of the tantalizing benefits of an active lifestyle, there's less and less chance you'll revert back to your unhealthy inactivity.

Exercise dropout rate

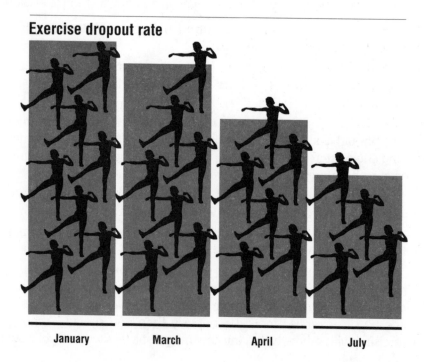

January	March	April	July

Table 4.1
Walking Health Points Chart

Time (min:sec)	Distance (miles)	Health points	Time (min:sec)	Distance (miles)	Health points
5:00	Under 0.10	0.8	7:30	Under 0.15	1.3
	0.10-0.14	1.0		0.15-0.19	1.5
	0.15-0.19	1.2		0.20-0.24	1.7
	0.20-0.24	1.4		0.25-0.29	1.9
	0.25-0.29	1.6		0.30-0.34	2.1
	0.30-0.33	1.8		0.35-0.39	2.3
	Over 0.33	*		0.40-0.44	2.5
				0.45-0.49	2.7
				Over 0.49	*
10:00	Under 0.20	1.7	12:30	Under 0.20	1.9
	0.20-0.24	1.8		0.20-0.29	2.3
	0.25-0.29	2.0		0.30-0.39	2.7
	0.30-0.34	2.2		0.40-0.49	3.1
	0.35-0.39	2.4		0.50-0.59	3.5
	0.40-0.44	2.6		0.60-0.69	3.9
	0.45-0.49	2.8		0.70-0.79	4.3
	0.50-0.54	3.0		0.80-0.83	4.7
	0.55-0.59	3.2		Over 0.83	*
	0.60-0.66	3.6			
	Over 0.66	*			
15:00	Under 0.30	2.5	17:30	Under 0.30	2.8
	0.30-0.39	2.9		0.30-0.49	3.5
	0.40-0.49	3.3		0.50-0.69	4.3
	0.50-0.59	3.7		0.70-0.89	5.1
	0.60-0.69	4.1		0.90-1.09	5.9
	0.70-0.79	4.5		1.10-1.16	6.7
	0.80-0.89	4.9		Over 1.16	*
	0.90-0.99	5.3			
	Over 0.99	*			
20:00	Under 0.40	3.4	22:30	Under 0.40	3.6
	0.40-0.59	4.1		0.40-0.59	4.4
	0.60-0.79	4.9		0.60-0.79	5.2
	0.80-0.99	5.7		0.80-0.99	6.0
	1.00-1.19	6.5		1.00-1.19	6.8
	1.20-1.33	7.3		1.20-1.39	7.6
	Over 1.33	*		1.40-1.49	8.4
				Over 1.49	*
25:00	Under 0.50	4.2	27:30	Under 0.50	4.5
	0.50-0.69	5.0		0.50-0.69	5.2
	0.70-0.89	5.8		0.70-0.89	6.0

(Cont.)

Table 4.1
(Continued)

Time (min:sec)	Distance (miles)	Health points	Time (min:sec)	Distance (miles)	Health points
25:00 (Cont.)			27:30 (Cont.)		
	0.90-1.09	6.6		0.90-1.09	6.8
	1.10-1.29	7.4		1.10-1.29	7.6
	1.30-1.49	8.2		1.30-1.49	8.4
	1.50-1.66	9.0		1.50-1.69	9.2
	Over 1.66	*		1.70-1.83	10.0
				Over 1.83	*
30:00	Under 0.50	4.6	35:00	Under 0.75	6.1
	0.50-0.74	5.6		0.75-0.99	7.0
	0.75-0.99	6.6		1.00-1.24	8.0
	1.00-1.24	7.6		1.25-1.49	9.0
	1.25-1.49	8.6		1.50-1.74	10.0
	1.50-1.74	9.6		1.75-1.99	11.0
	1.75-1.99	10.6		2.00-2.24	12.0
	Over 1.99	*		2.25-2.33	13.0
				Over 2.33	*
40:00	Under 1.00	7.5	45:00	Under 1.00	7.9
	1.00-1.24	8.5		1.00-1.49	9.9
	1.25-1.49	9.5		1.50-1.99	11.9
	1.50-1.74	10.5		2.00-2.49	13.9
	1.75-1.99	11.5		2.50-2.99	15.9
	2.00-2.24	12.5		Over 2.99	*
	2.25-2.49	13.5			
	2.50-2.66	14.5			
	Over 2.66	*			
50:00	Under 1.00	8.4	55:00	Under 1.00	8.8
	1.00-1.49	10.3		1.00-1.49	10.8
	1.50-1.99	12.4		1.50-1.99	12.8
	2.00-2.49	14.4		2.00-2.49	14.8
	2.50-2.99	16.4		2.50-2.99	16.8
	3.00-3.33	18.4		3.00-3.49	18.8
	Over 3.33	*		3.50-3.66	20.8
				Over 3.66	*
60:00	Under 1.00	9.3			
	1.00-1.49	11.2			
	1.50-1.99	13.2			
	2.00-2.49	15.2			
	2.50-2.99	17.2			
	3.00-3.49	19.2			
	3.50-3.99	21.2			
	Over 3.99	*			

*Use the Jogging Health Points Chart (Table 4.2).

Table 4.2
Jogging Health Points Chart

Time (min:sec)	Distance (miles)	Health points	Time (min:sec)	Distance (miles)	Health points
5:00	Under 0.40	3.6	7:30	Under 0.50	4.7
	0.40-0.49	4.4		0.50-0.59	5.4
	0.50-0.59	5.2		0.60-0.69	6.2
	0.60-0.69	6.0		0.70-0.79	7.0
	Over 0.69	6.8		0.80-0.89	7.8
				0.90-0.99	8.6
				1.00-1.09	9.4
				Over 1.09	10.2
10:00	Under 0.80	7.3	12:30	Under 1.00	9.2
	0.80-0.89	8.0		1.00-1.19	10.7
	0.90-0.99	8.8		1.20-1.39	12.3
	1.00-1.09	9.6		1.40-1.59	13.9
	1.10-1.19	10.4		1.60-1.79	15.5
	1.20-1.29	11.2		Over 1.79	17.1
	1.30-1.39	12.0			
	1.40-1.49	12.8			
	Over 1.49	13.6			
15:00	Under 1.20	10.9	17:30	Under 1.40	12.8
	1.20-1.39	12.5		1.40-1.59	14.3
	1.40-1.59	14.1		1.60-1.79	15.9
	1.60-1.79	15.7		1.80-1.99	17.5
	1.80-1.99	17.3		2.00-2.19	19.1
	2.00-2.19	18.9		2.20-2.39	20.7
	Over 2.19	20.5		2.40-2.59	22.4
				Over 2.59	24.0
20:00	Under 1.50	13.8	22:30	Under 1.75	16.0
	1.50-1.74	15.7		1.75-1.99	18.0
	1.75-1.99	17.7		2.00-2.24	20.0
	2.00-2.24	19.7		2.25-2.49	22.0
	2.25-2.49	21.7		2.50-2.74	24.0
	2.50-2.74	23.7		2.75-2.99	26.0
	2.75-2.99	25.7		3.00-3.24	28.0
	Over 2.99	27.7		Over 3.24	30.0
25:00	Under 2.00	18.2	27:30	Under 2.00	18.5
	2.00-2.24	20.2		2.00-2.24	20.4
	2.25-2.49	22.2		2.25-2.49	22.4
	2.50-2.74	24.2		2.50-2.74	24.4
	2.75-2.99	26.2		2.75-2.99	26.4
	3.00-3.24	28.2		3.00-3.24	28.4
	3.25-3.49	30.2		3.25-3.49	30.4
	3.50-3.74	32.2		3.50-3.74	32.5

(Cont.)

Table 4.2
(Continued)

Time (min:sec)	Distance (miles)	Health points	Time (min:sec)	Distance (miles)	Health points
25:00 (Cont.)			27:30 (Cont.)		
	Over 3.74	34.2		3.75-3.99	34.5
				Over 3.99	36.5
30:00	Under 2.50	22.7	35:00	Under 2.75	25.1
	2.50-2.74	24.6		2.75-2.99	27.0
	2.75-2.99	26.6		3.00-3.24	29.1
	3.00-3.24	28.6		3.25-3.49	31.1
	3.25-3.49	30.6		3.50-3.74	33.1
	3.50-3.74	32.6		3.75-3.99	35.1
	3.75-3.99	34.6		4.00-4.24	37.1
	4.00-4.24	36.6		4.25-4.49	39.1
	Over 4.24	38.6		4.50-4.74	41.1
				4.75-4.99	43.1
				Over 4.99	45.1
40:00	Under 3.00	27.6	45:00	Under 3.50	32.0
	3.00-3.49	31.5		3.50-3.99	35.9
	3.50-3.99	35.5		4.00-4.49	40.0
	4.00-4.49	39.5		4.50-4.99	44.0
	4.50-4.99	43.5		5.00-5.49	48.0
	5.00-5.49	47.5		5.50-5.99	52.0
	5.50-5.99	51.6		6.00-6.49	56.0
	Over 5.99	55.6		Over 6.49	60.0
50:00	Under 4.00	36.5	55:00	Under 4.50	40.9
	4.00-4.49	40.4		4.50-4.99	44.8
	4.50-4.99	44.4		5.00-5.49	48.9
	5.00-5.49	48.4		5.50-5.99	52.9
	5.50-5.99	52.4		6.00-6.49	56.9
	6.00-6.49	56.4		6.50-6.99	60.9
	6.50-6.99	60.4		7.00-7.49	64.9
	7.00-7.49	64.5		7.50-7.99	68.9
	Over 7.49	68.5		Over 7.99	72.9
60:00	Under 4.50	41.3			
	4.50-4.99	45.3			
	5.00-5.49	49.3			
	5.50-5.99	53.3			
	6.00-6.49	57.3			
	6.50-6.99	61.3			
	7.00-7.49	65.3			
	7.50-7.99	69.3			
	8.00-8.49	73.4			
	8.50-8.99	77.4			
	Over 8.99	81.4			

Table 4.3
Stationary Cycling (Legs Only) Health Points Chart

	Health points per minute							
Work rate (watts)	Under 100 lb	100 to 124 lb	125 to 149 lb	150 to 174 lb	175 to 199 lb	200 to 224 lb	225 to 249 lb	Over 249 lb
Under 25	0.34	0.28	0.24	0.22	0.20	0.18	0.17	0.16
25-49	0.54	0.44	0.36	0.32	0.28	0.26	0.24	0.22
50-74	0.76	0.60	0.50	0.42	0.38	0.34	0.32	0.30
75-99	0.98	0.76	0.62	0.54	0.48	0.42	0.38	0.36
100-124	1.20	0.92	0.76	0.64	0.56	0.50	0.46	0.42
125-149	1.42	1.10	0.90	0.76	0.66	0.58	0.54	0.48
150-174	1.64	1.26	1.02	0.86	0.76	0.68	0.60	0.56
175-199	1.86	1.42	1.16	0.98	0.84	0.76	0.68	0.62
200-224	2.08	1.58	1.28	1.08	0.94	0.84	0.76	0.68
225-249	2.30	1.76	1.42	1.20	1.04	0.92	0.82	0.76
Over 249	2.52	1.92	1.56	1.30	1.14	1.00	0.90	0.82

Table 4.4
Schwinn Air-Dyne Health Points Chart

	Health points per minute							
Work load	Under 100 lb	100 to 124 lb	125 to 149 lb	150 to 174 lb	175 to 199 lb	200 to 224 lb	225 to 249 lb	Over 249 lb
Under 0.5	0.34	0.28	0.24	0.22	0.20	0.18	0.17	0.16
0.5-0.9	0.52	0.40	0.34	0.30	0.26	0.24	0.22	0.21
1.0-1.4	0.74	0.56	0.48	0.40	0.36	0.32	0.30	0.28
1.5-1.9	0.96	0.74	0.60	0.52	0.46	0.42	0.38	0.34
2.0-2.4	1.18	0.90	0.74	0.62	0.56	0.50	0.44	0.42
2.5-2.9	1.40	1.06	0.86	0.74	0.64	0.58	0.52	0.48
3.0-3.4	1.62	1.22	1.00	0.84	0.74	0.66	0.60	0.54
3.5-3.9	1.84	1.40	1.14	0.96	0.84	0.74	0.66	0.62
4.0-4.4	2.06	1.56	1.26	1.06	0.92	0.82	0.74	0.68
4.5-4.9	2.28	1.72	1.40	1.18	1.02	0.90	0.82	0.74
Over 4.9	2.50	1.88	1.52	1.28	1.12	0.98	0.88	0.80

Table 4.5
Other Aerobic Activities

	Health points per minute		
		Intensity*	
Activity	Light	Moderate	Heavy
Aerobic dancing	0.35	0.53	0.79
Alpine skiing	0.35	0.53	0.70
Aqua-aerobics	0.35	0.53	0.79
Arm-cycle ergometry	0.22	0.35	0.61
Backpacking	0.53	0.70	0.88
(5% slope, 44 lbs or 20 kg)			
4.0 mph (6.4 kph)	0.70		
4.5 mph (7.2 kph)	0.84		
5.0 mph (8.0 kph)	1.02		
6.0 mph (9.6 kph)	1.15		
7.0 mph (11.2 kph)	1.36		
Badminton	0.26	0.53	0.79
Ballet	0.44	0.53	0.70
Ballroom dancing	0.26	0.35	0.44
Baseball	0.26	0.35	0.44
Basketball	0.53	0.70	0.96
Bicycling	0.26	0.61	0.88
6.3 mph (10 kph)	0.42		
9.4 mph (15 kph)	0.52		
12.5 mph (10 kph)	0.62		
15.6 mph (25 kph)	0.74		
18.8 mph (30 kph)	0.86		
Canoeing	0.26	0.35	0.53
Catch (ball)	0.26	0.35	0.44
Circuit resistance training	0.26	0.44	0.61
Cricket	0.26	0.35	0.44
Cross-country skiing	0.44	0.79	1.14
2.5 mph (4 kph)	0.48		
3.8 mph (6 kph)	0.67		
5.0 mph (8 kph)	0.87		
6.3 mph (10 kph)	1.07		
7.5 mph (12 kph)	1.25		
8.8 mph (14 kph)	1.44		
Exercise classes	0.35	0.53	0.79
Fencing	0.44	0.61	0.88
Field hockey	0.53	0.70	0.88
Figure skating	0.35	0.53	0.88

| Activity | Health points per minute | | |
| | Intensity* | | |
	Light	Moderate	Heavy
Football (American)		0.44	0.53	0.61
Football (touch)		0.44	0.53	0.70
Golf				
Carrying clubs	0.45			
Pulling cart	0.35			
Riding cart	0.22			
Gymnastics		0.44	0.61	0.88
Handball (4-wall)		0.53	0.70	0.96
Hiking		0.26	0.53	0.70
Home calisthenics		0.26	0.44	0.70
Hunting		0.26	0.44	0.61
Ice hockey		0.53	0.70	0.88
Judo		0.53	0.70	1.05
Karate		0.44	0.70	1.05
Kayaking		0.53	0.70	0.96
7.8 mph (12.5 kph)	0.68			
9.4 mph (15.0 kph)	0.96			
Lacrosse		0.53	0.70	0.88
Modern dancing		0.44	0.53	0.70
Mountaineering		0.61	0.70	0.88
Orienteering		0.70	0.88	1.05
Racquetball		0.53	0.79	1.05
Rebounding		0.31	0.44	0.53
Rollerskating		0.44	0.57	0.70
Rope skipping		0.61	0.88	1.05
66 per min	0.86			
84 per min	0.92			
100 per min	0.96			
120 per min	1.00			
125 per min	1.02			
130 per min	1.03			
135 per min	1.05			
145 per min	1.06			
Rowing		0.61	0.88	1.14
2.5 mph (4 kph)	0.48			
5.0 mph (8 kph)	0.90			
7.5 mph (12 kph)	1.18			
10.0 mph (16 kph)	1.44			

(Cont.)

Table 4.5
(Continued)

| Activity | Health points per minute | | |
| | Intensity* | | |
	Light	Moderate	Heavy
Rowing (Cont.)			
12.5 mph (20 kph)	1.67		
Rugby		0.53	0.70	0.96
Scuba diving		0.35	0.44	0.53
Sculling		0.35	0.53	0.88
Skateboarding		0.44	0.57	0.70
Skating (ice)		0.35	0.61	1.14
11.3 mph (18 kph)	0.35		
15.6 mph (25 kph)	0.42		
17.5 mph (28 kph)	0.81		
20.0 mph (32 kph)	0.95		
22.5 mph (36 kph)	1.33		
Snorkeling		0.35	0.44	0.53
Soccer		0.44	0.61	0.96
Softball		0.26	0.35	0.44
Squash		0.53	0.79	1.05
Stair climbing		0.35	0.61	0.96
Swimming (beach)		0.18	0.26	0.35
Swimming (pool)		0.26	0.44	0.79
1.3 mph (2 kph)	0.38		
1.6 mph (2.5 kph)	0.60		
1.9 mph (3.0 kph)	0.78		
2.2 mph (3.5 kph)	1.01		
2.5 mph (4.0 kph)	1.19		
Synchronized swimming		0.35	0.53	0.70
Table tennis		0.26	0.44	0.70
Tennis		0.35	0.53	0.88
Volleyball		0.44	0.53	0.70
Walking up stairs		0.35	0.53	0.70
Water polo		0.53	0.70	0.96
Wrestling		0.53	0.79	1.05

*Light intensity results in minimal perspiration and only a slight increase in breathing above normal (RPE of less than 12). Moderate intensity results in definite perspiration and above normal breathing (RPE of 12-13). Heavy intensity corresponds to heavy perspiration and breathing (RPE of more than 13). These values are adapted from an expert committee report of the Canada Fitness Survey - source M. Jette et al., Clinical Cardiology, 13 (1990): 555-565.

Chapter 4
Prescription

☐ If you're a novice exerciser, consider using one of my beginning exercise programs (see chapter 3). Let your doctor help you adapt it to suit the medical realities of your particular case of CFS.

☐ Use our Health Points System to gain optimal health benefits with minimal risk.

☐ When using our Health Points System, modulate your frequency, intensity, and duration of exercise to earn 50 to 100 points each week.

☐ Do not attempt to earn your quota of health points in fewer than 3 workouts—on at least 3 separate days—each week.

☐ Keep your goals realistic and modify them continually as your condition changes.

☐ If your condition is such that you cannot attain the desired weekly number of health points, don't become discouraged. Provided you perform some type of aerobic exercise for a minimum of 15 minutes at least 3 days a week, you'll derive important health benefits.

☐ Be proud of whatever progress you are able to make.

☐ Do everything in your power to keep from becoming an exercise dropout, especially during the crucial initial months.

Chapter 5

Staying Within the Safe-Exercise Zone: Essential Guidelines for People With CFS

Fortunately, much of the guesswork has been eliminated from the process of prescribing exercise as a means of improving general health and fitness. Today, well-informed physicians can prescribe exercise just as they would a medication. But, just as with drugs, certain precautions are in order to make sure your exercise regimen is both safe and effective.

People of any health status should adhere to certain general safety guidelines in an exercise program. All of these are detailed in other books from the Cooper Clinic, such as *Running Without Fear*,[1] *The Aerobics Program for Total Well-Being*,[2] and *The New Aerobics for Women*,[3] so I won't repeat them here. Rather, I want to focus on the special problems and hazards associated with exercise for CFS patients.

SIX SAFE-EXERCISE GUIDELINES

The safety guidelines I outline are intended to reduce the chances that you'll develop any exercise-related cardiac complications, musculo-skeletal injuries, or a worsening of your chronic fatigue and other CFS symptoms. I urge you to follow them as well as listen to the advice of your doctor.

EXERCISE SAFETY GUIDELINE 1

Have a thorough medical evaluation before starting your exercise program—and at regular intervals thereafter.

Any CFS patient should undergo a complete medical exam (see Appendix C) and get a doctor's permission before embarking on an exercise program. The primary purpose of this comprehensive checkup is to insure that there isn't a potentially treatable cause for your chronic fatigue or any conditions that may be worsened by exercise, even appropriately performed.[4,5] Specifically, expect your doctor to withhold permission if you have any of the following conditions, which place aerobic exercise completely off limits, at least for now.

✓ Do *NOT* Exercise if Your Physician Indicates You Have Any ✓ of These Conditions

_____ Unstable angina pectoris or a recent severe heart attack

_____ Recent significant change in resting ECG that has not been adequately investigated and managed

_____ A recent embolism

_____ Thrombophlebitis or an intracardiac thrombus

_____ Active or suspected myocarditis or pericarditis

_____ Acute or inadequately controlled heart failure

_____ Moderate to severe aortic stenosis

_____ Clinically significant hypertrophic obstructive cardiomyopathy

_____ Suspected or known aneurysm, cardiac or vascular, that your doctor feels may be worsened by exercise

_____ Uncontrolled atrial or ventricular arrhythmias that are considered clinically significant

_____ Resting heart rate higher than 100 beats per minute that has not been fully investigated

_____ Third-degree heart block

_____ Uncontrolled hypertension with resting systolic blood pressure above 200 mmHg or diastolic blood pressure above 120 mmHg

_____ Recent fall in systolic blood pressure of more than 20 mmHg that was not caused by medication

_____ Uncontrolled metabolic disease, such as diabetes mellitus, thyrotoxicosis, or myxedema

_____ Acute infection

_____ Oral temperature 99.5 °F (37.5 °C) or above

_____ Chronic infectious disease such as hepatitis or AIDS that your doctor feels may be worsened by exercise

_____ Significant electrolyte disturbances

_____ Neuromuscular, musculoskeletal, or rheumatoid disorders that your doctor thinks exercise may exacerbate

_____ Pregnancy complications

_____ Major emotional distress (psychosis)

_____ Any other condition known to preclude exercise

Note. From American College of Sports Medicine: Guidelines for Exercise Testing and Prescription, 4th edition. Philadelphia, Lea and Febiger, 1991. Adapted with permission of the publisher.

Of course, your pre-exercise medical exam won't be your last. While you continue to manifest symptoms of CFS, you should be reevaluated every 4 to 6 months to insure that your CFS is not a result of some previously undetected illness and that exercise is not worsening your condition. Shorten the interval between checkups even more should your symptoms worsen or new ones develop.

I'm a great proponent of exercise testing. All our CFS patients about to start an exercise program take a "symptom-limited maximal exercise test" with electrocardiogram and blood pressure monitoring.

Not only does this test let us screen for cardiac abnormalities, but it's also a guide to how much aerobic exercise a patient will be able to do initially and a way to measure maximal heart rate. With this information we can tailor an aerobic exercise program to each patient's specific condition. This same information will be useful to you in undertaking the exercise program outlined in this book; thus, I urge you to have a pretest if at all possible. After 3 to 6 months of regular exercise, your fitness level and possibly your maximal heart rate are likely to have improved substantially. Another test at this point will better enable you to monitor the effectiveness of your exertion. Thereafter, it's probably only necessary to repeat this test once a year for safety reasons and to assess your progress.

EXERCISE SAFETY GUIDELINE 2

Find out whether you need direct medical supervision when you exercise—and whether it's needed permanently or only during the early weeks of the program.

Just about every person with CFS is capable of doing carefully tailored stretching and muscle-strengthening exercises. But for some CFS patients, aerobic exercise may be too risky. For other CFS patients, aerobic exercise may be possible—*but only under special supervised conditions.* In a "medically supervised" exercise program, a doctor or other qualified health professional—such as a physical therapist, exercise physiologist, or nurse—is present overseeing the exercise. Your doctor should be able to refer you to such a program in your area. A cardiac rehabilitation program is a good choice because the staff is also equipped to monitor patients, like you, with other special medical needs.

If you check off any of the following circumstances, you should err in the direction of caution and begin exercising in a supervised program at least for the first 12 weeks.

 ## Conditions That Require
Supervised Exercise

_____ I'm severely impaired or debilitated by my CFS (see chapter 2).

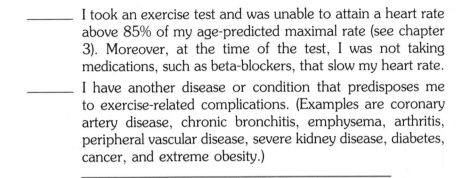

_____ I took an exercise test and was unable to attain a heart rate above 85% of my age-predicted maximal rate (see chapter 3). Moreover, at the time of the test, I was not taking medications, such as beta-blockers, that slow my heart rate.

_____ I have another disease or condition that predisposes me to exercise-related complications. (Examples are coronary artery disease, chronic bronchitis, emphysema, arthritis, peripheral vascular disease, severe kidney disease, diabetes, cancer, and extreme obesity.)

If you are predisposed to exercise-related complications, you may need to exercise under medical supervision indefinitely. On the other hand, even if none of the circumstances listed apply to you, you still require medically directed exercise, with your physician aware of your regimen and periodically evaluating your organic response, making changes in your program where necessary.

DRUG ALERT FOR CFS PATIENTS

Ask your doctor if any medications you're taking put you at greater risk during exercise—or alter your heart rate's response to exertion.

EXERCISE SAFETY GUIDELINE 3

Know the warning signs of an impending cardiac problem.

The information I'm giving you about exercise safety is not meant to scare you away. The fact remains that exercise is a far more normal state of human affairs than indolence and it can be done with a great degree of confidence by the vast majority of people with CFS.

What it comes down to is this: You're probably far more likely to die from the deleterious effects of sedentary living than you are to suffer from sudden death during exercise. On the other hand, it's still prudent to keep your risk as low as reasonably possible. One of the best ways to boost your risk-to-benefit ratio is to remember this axiom:

Although death during exercise is always unexpected, it's seldom unheralded.

In other words, in many instances, you'll have some warning that things are awry. This box lists the bodily signs indicating that all might not be well with your heart. Should you experience any of them before, during, or just after your exercise sessions, discuss them with your doctor before continuing with exercise.

WARNING SIGNS OF HEART PROBLEMS

✓ *Pain or discomfort in your chest, abdomen, back, neck, jaw, or arms.* Such symptoms may be signs of an inadequate supply of blood and oxygen to your heart muscle because of potentially serious conditions such as atherosclerotic plaque buildup in your coronary arteries.

✓ *A nauseous sensation during or after exercise.* This can result from a variety of causes, but it can also signify a cardiac abnormality.

✓ *Unaccustomed shortness of breath during exercise.* Any kind of aerobic exercise may make you huff and puff. This isn't what I'm referring to here. Let's say an ordinary part of your routine is to walk 2 miles in 35 minutes with no breathlessness. If one day you can't do it anymore, you should be alarmed.

✓ *Dizziness or fainting.* This can occur in perfectly healthy people who don't follow proper exercise protocol and fail to cool down adequately. Anyone could feel dizzy momentarily or even actually faint if he or she stops exercising suddenly. The type of dizziness I'm concerned about occurs *while* you're exercising rather than upon stopping suddenly. This is a more probable sign of a serious heart problem and warrants immediate medical consultation.

✓ *An irregular pulse, particularly when it's been regular in your past exercise sessions.* If you notice what appears to be extra heartbeats or skipped beats, notify your doctor. This too might not be anything of significance; on the other hand, it could point to heart problems.

✓ *A very rapid heart rate at rest.* This means 100 beats per minute or higher after at least 5 minutes of rest. Although this could result from a variety of causes, including a fever, it can also point to cardiac abnormalities. It should be reported to your doctor.

EXERCISE SAFETY GUIDELINE 4

Put safety at the top of your exercise priority list by following proper exercise protocol.

When it comes to exercise, there's a right way and a wrong way to do it, a safe way and a dangerous way. Even healthy people who exercise should adhere to certain general safety guidelines, all of which have been described in detail in other books from the Cooper Clinic. These I include here have special relevance for exercisers with CFS:

• *Warm up and cool down adequately—a minimum of five minutes for each.* Sufficient warm-up and cool-down are important for every exerciser because over 70% of all cardiac problems that surface during exercise do so either at the beginning or end of a session. Also, warming up may reduce your risk for musculoskeletal injuries.

Adequate warm-up and cool-down are especially important for people with CFS, according to a Canadian study, which suggests that the heart rates of some CFS patients respond more slowly to changes in exercise intensity than the heart rates of healthy individuals.[6]

• *Don't exercise in adverse climatic conditions, particularly without taking adequate precautions.* Hyperthermia—an overheating of the body during exercise—impairs your ability to exercise and predisposes you to heat stroke, a potentially fatal condition. CFS

Symptoms of hyperthermia

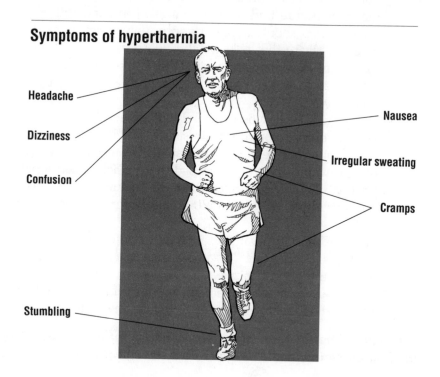

Headache

Dizziness

Confusion

Stumbling

Nausea

Irregular sweating

Cramps

patients who exercise when their temperatures are slightly above normal should be aware of their increased risk for exercise-induced hyperthermia.

The symptoms of hyperthermia include headache, dizziness, confusion, stumbling, nausea, cramps, and cessation of sweating or excessive sweating.

To avoid hyperthermia, here are four preventive measures you can take:

—If you're exercising outdoors, let weather conditions be your guide to the amount and intensity of exercise you should indulge in on a given day. When heat and humidity are high, be sensible. Don't engage in strenuous exercise. When it's hot and humid we monitor the wet bulb globe temperature (WBGT) index at The Cooper Aerobics Center to decide when our exercisers should be cautioned either to moderate their efforts or not exercise outdoors at all. The WBGT index is calculated from the readings of 3 types of thermometers. They measure humidity, radiant heat, and air temperature. If you don't have access to the WBGT index, the temperature-humidity chart shown in Figure 5.1 can be substituted. When the temperature and humidity intersect in zones other than Zone 1, you should take the appropriate precautions. Likewise, be aware that cold weather worsens the usual disease symptoms in some people with CFS. If this is so for you, you may need to modify your exercise program accordingly on such days.

—Drink fluids while you're exercising, especially on hot days. Do this even if you're not thirsty. About 15 minutes before you begin your session, drink about 8 ounces (or 240 ml) of cold water, which is absorbed more quickly than tepid. If your workout lasts longer than 30 minutes, take another 8-ounce drink at 15- to 20-minute intervals during exercise.

—When exercising in warm weather, wear clothing that promotes heat loss. Fabrics that "breathe," such as a mesh or "fishnet" T-shirt, are good choices.

—If you must exercise in the heat, sponge off the exposed parts of your body with cool water at regular intervals.

• *Skip exercise when you have a fever, influenza, or other moderately serious acute illness.* CFS is sometimes accompanied by

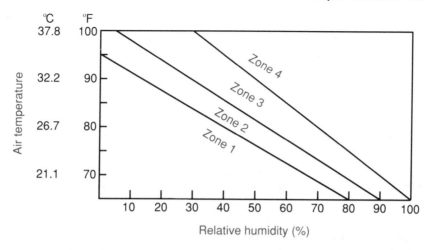

Zone 1: Feel free to engage in unrestricted outdoor exercise. WBGT index is less than 85°F.
Zone 2: Restrict your exercise unless you've been working out in similar conditions for a period of at least 10 days. WBGT index is between 85 and 87°F. Cardiac patients should limit outdoor exercise to a maximum of 45 minutes, even if acclimatized.
Zone 3: Severely restrict your exercise unless you've been working out in similar conditions for a period of at least 30 days. WBGT index is between 88 and 90°F. Cardiac patients should limit outdoor exercise to maximum of 30 minutes, even if acclimatized.
Zone 4: Stay indoors and turn on the air conditioner. Don't even contemplate outdoor exertion on a day like this. WBGT index is more than 90°F.

Figure 5.1   Temperature-humidity chart.

a chronic mild fever. It can result from a variety of conditions, one of which is active viral infection. If you suffer from intermittent fevers, or if your CFS was preceded by an acute viral illness, it's a good idea to take your temperature before each workout.

In view of my warning about viral myocarditis in chapter 2 (see page 23), I think it's imprudent to undertake a vigorous aerobic workout when your oral temperature is 99.5 °F (37.5 °C) or above. On the other hand, if your temperature is 99.5 °F or above but below 100.4 °F (or 38 °C), you can perform *gentle* stretching and isometric muscle-strengthening exercises such as those in chapter 3 if you feel up to it.

Acute illnesses usually subside on their own after a relatively short time or can be cured. If you've got nothing more serious than a cold, go ahead with aerobics if your temperature is normal, your symptoms are above your neck (for example, runny nose, sneezing, scratchy throat) and you feel like it. But when your acute ailment is more serious—and especially if it's accompanied by fever—sit out all forms of strenuous exercise until you're better.[7] After an illness, ease back into aerobics gradually over the course of at least a week or two.

• *Take the necessary steps to reduce your risk for orthopedic injuries.* Common sense is the key to avoiding exercise-induced musculoskeletal injuries. Don't attempt to make up for lost months or years of sedentary living overnight by starting off like gangbusters. Rather, take it slow and easy in the beginning as I outline in chapter 3.

To limber up your body before exertion, stretch before each exercise session; whenever possible, stretch at the end of each session, too. Moreover, if you choose a high-impact, weight-bearing exercise such as jogging, use your head: Don't do it day after day on hard surfaces; ease the impact by doing it on grass or some other cushioned surface at least part of the time.

The right shoes are crucial for every exerciser who wants to avoid foot and knee problems and other injuries. Because of recent technological advances there are shoes specially designed for particular weight-bearing activities and they are engineered to suit different types of feet. A qualified health professional is the best source of information about shoes to meet your particular needs. I'd also suggest that you patronize a quality shoe store where the sales staff are knowledgeable about athletic footgear. If you're a jogger, consult the periodic shoe evaluations that appear in the various runners' magazines. These consumer guides give you a look at the choices in various categories of athletic footgear and highlight what to seek out and what to avoid.

EXERCISE SAFETY GUIDELINE 5

Closely monitor your body's response to exercise to make sure you're not overdoing it. Be aware of the warning signs of over-training—the condition where your workouts no longer benefit you.

In other words, *stay in tune with your body.* This is critical because in some people CFS tends to wax and wane. In periods of remission, you may think you're permanently rid of your lassitude, only to be disappointed when a flare-up forces you to cut back drastically on your exercise regimen. You may make the mistake of overdoing it during those periods when your body seems miraculously restored to health. Or you may be like some of our CFS patients—impatient, competitive, driven people determined to fight their malady with every weapon they possess. A strong, indomitable will makes them overdo their exercise program to the point of overtraining.

The warning indicators of overtraining are well-known to doctors of sports medicine who work with competitive athletes.[8] Here's a checklist of typical overtraining signs, many of which are similar to CFS's symptoms.[9]

✓   Signs of Overtraining   ✓

_____ Changes in sleep patterns, especially newfound insomnia

_____ Longer healing period for minor cuts and scratches

_____ Fall in blood pressure and dizziness when getting up from a prone or seated position

_____ Gastrointestinal disturbances, especially diarrhea

_____ Gradual loss of weight in the absence of dieting or increased physical activity

_____ Greater than usual increase in heart rate during a standard exercise session

_____ Leaden or sluggish feeling in legs during exercise

_____ Impaired mental acuity and performance or inability to concentrate

_____ Inability to complete routine exercise training sessions that were no special challenge before

_____ Increase in your resting heart rate (recorded early in the morning) by more than 10 beats per minute

_____ Excessive thirst and fluid consumption at night

_____ Greater susceptibility to infections, allergies, headaches, and injury

_____ Lethargy, listlessness, and tiredness

_____ Loss of appetite

(Cont.)

_____ General loss of enthusiasm, drive, and motivation. In athletes or other people who usually derive joy from exercise, this disinterest and lack of incentive extends to this sphere as well.

_____ Loss of libido or interest in sex

_____ Irregular or no menstruation in premenopausal women

_____ Muscle and joint pains

_____ Sluggishness that persists for more than 24 hours after a workout

_____ Swelling of the lymph nodes

Should you suspect that overtraining is your problem, you may need to cut back on your exercise schedule. On the other hand, it's unwise to jump to such conclusions during the first few weeks after you begin an exercise program. I find my novice CFS exercisers often misinterpret what are actually normal reactions to exertion as signs of overtraining. They're anxious about their condition and so attuned to their own adverse symptoms that they assume that any new bodily response that's even slightly negative is something to worry about. If you are unsure whether you've been overtraining, a discussion with your doctor should help you decide.

Let's face it, not all the feelings associated with exercise are pleasant. Exertion speeds up your heart rate, which can be frightening to people who aren't used to it. Your breathing becomes faster, deeper, and more labored, and you start to sweat. If you continue doing an endurance exercise long enough, your muscles eventually tire. But once you slow down or stop completely, these feelings begin to subside.

You may find that your muscles feel a little sore the next day and even somewhat weaker than usual. This is called "delayed-onset muscle soreness" and is perfectly natural. It can persist for up to 10 days after you've started a type of exercise using muscles unaccustomed to strenuous use.[10] Delayed soreness is nothing to worry about unless it's terribly severe. Recent studies show that continuing to exercise despite some soreness poses little or no risk. In fact, after each subsequent exercise session, you should find the soreness abating as your muscles adapt to your new habitual movements.[11] Within a matter of weeks, the soreness should be gone completely or hardly noticeable.

EXERCISE SAFETY GUIDELINE 6

Never ignore a trend indicating that your symptoms are getting worse.

Although exercise training is by no means a panacea for CFS, you can rest assured that faithful adherence to the Health Points program outlined in chapter 4 should increase your fitness substantially with minimum risk. On the other hand, no two people with CFS respond to exercise in exactly the same way. I've known a few CFS patients who have had to give up on serious aerobic exercise. Before I concur with such a decision, however, I make sure our patients have given exercise a fair trial; in my view, this means at least 12 weeks. I also make sure they have followed all my safety guidelines to the letter.

Should you be one of the few unfortunate CFS patients who find themselves in this category, I recommend that you face reality after 12 solid weeks of trying conscientiously and discuss with your doctor what role, if any, aerobic exercise should play in your treatment and rehabilitation program.

One way to track the long-term course of your condition is to use both of the CFS symptom monitoring systems that follow. Make photocopies of both systems and fill them in weekly.

The first is a Chronic Fatigue Scorecard. Each week, I encourage you to take this short four-question test, referred to as the Rand Index of Vitality.[12] The lower your score, the more severe your chronic fatigue; the higher your score, the better off you are. After a number of weeks filling in the scorecard, if you note a trend indicating a lessening of your fatigue, be happy and continue your current exercise program. If you detect a trend in the opposite direction, a change in your regimen is warranted.

I also recommend that you track the *overall* severity of your CFS—your fatigue as well as your other CFS symptoms—over time by filling in the CFS Symptom-Rating Scale (page 105) once a week.

Transfer the totals from the Chronic Fatigue Scorecard and the CFS Symptom-Rating Scale to the CFS Month-by-Month Symptom Overview (page 105). After a few months, patterns will begin to emerge, and you'll be able to see trends in the course of your disease at a glance.

104

Chronic Fatigue Scorecard:
This week, my score was _____.

1. **During the past week, I had energy, pep, and vitality to this degree:**
   - _____ (a) Very energetic, lots of pep   6
   - _____ (b) Fairly energetic most of the time   5
   - _____ (c) Energy level that varies quite a bit from day to day   4
   - _____ (d) Generally low in energy or pep most of the time   3
   - _____ (e) Very low in energy or pep most of the time   2
   - _____ (f) No energy or pep at all; I feel drained, sapped   1

2. **During the past week, I've felt tired, worn out, used up, or exhausted with this frequency:**
   - _____ (a) None of the time   6
   - _____ (b) A small portion of the time   5
   - _____ (c) Some of the time   4
   - _____ (d) A good bit of the time   3
   - _____ (e) Most of the time   2
   - _____ (f) All of the time   1

3. **During the past week, I've felt active and vigorous on the one extreme, and dull and sluggish on the other to the extent indicated below:**
   - _____ (a) Very active and vigorous every day   6
   - _____ (b) Mostly active and vigorous; never really dull or sluggish   5
   - _____ (c) Fairly active and vigorous; seldom dull or sluggish   4
   - _____ (d) Fairly dull or sluggish; seldom active or vigorous   3
   - _____ (e) Mostly dull or sluggish; never really active or vigorous   2
   - _____ (f) Very dull and sluggish every day   1

4. **During the past week, I've awakened feeling fresh and rested with this frequency:**
   - _____ (a) All of the time   6
   - _____ (b) Most of the time   5
   - _____ (c) A good bit of the time   4
   - _____ (d) Some of the time   3
   - _____ (e) A little of the time   2
   - _____ (f) None of the time   1

_____ **TOTAL** A score in the 1-14 range indicates abnormal fatigue.

Note. From A.F. Valdini, S. Steinhardt, J. Valicenti, A. Jaffe, "A One-Year Follow-up of Fatigued Patients," *The Journal of Family Practice*, 26:1, pp. 33-38. Copyright © 1988. Adapted by permission of Appleton & Lange, Inc.

CFS Symptom-Rating Scale

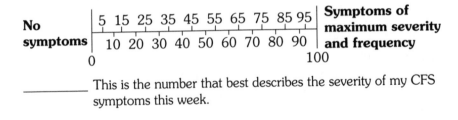

_____ This is the number that best describes the severity of my CFS symptoms this week.

CFS Month-by-Month Symptom Overview

Transfer the totals from your Chronic Fatigue Scorecard and CFS Symptom-Rating Scale to the corresponding boxes below.

	Jan.	Feb.	March	April	May	June	July	Aug.	Sept.	Oct.	Nov.	Dec.
Chronic Fatigue Scorecard:												
Week 1 total	—	—	—	—	—	—	—	—	—	—	—	—
Week 2 total	—	—	—	—	—	—	—	—	—	—	—	—
Week 3 total	—	—	—	—	—	—	—	—	—	—	—	—
Week 4 total	—	—	—	—	—	—	—	—	—	—	—	—
Total for month	═	═	═	═	═	═	═	═	═	═	═	═
CFS Symptom-Rating Scale:												
Week 1 rating	—	—	—	—	—	—	—	—	—	—	—	—
Week 2 rating	—	—	—	—	—	—	—	—	—	—	—	—
Week 3 rating	—	—	—	—	—	—	—	—	—	—	—	—
Week 4 rating	—	—	—	—	—	—	—	—	—	—	—	—
Total for month	═	═	═	═	═	═	═	═	═	═	═	═

SOME CONCLUDING THOUGHTS

In this book, I've offered you a state-of-the-art method for using regular exercise to reduce your fatigue and optimize both the quality and the quantity of your life. My advice has been based on what is currently known about exercise and CFS. In years to come, far more will certainly be learned about how CFS patients, such as yourself, can derive the most from an exercise rehabilitation program. But you shouldn't wait until then to exercise your options and embark on a physically active lifestyle. Now is the time for you, in consultation with your doctor, to formulate your specific game plan from the prototype I've provided.

The sooner you begin a sensible exercise program, the sooner you will reap the many rewards. Once you do get started, never forget that exercise should be fun. I've always enjoyed it thoroughly and have no doubt that with time you will too.

Good luck! And the best of health to you.

Chapter 5

Prescription

☐ Have a thorough medical evaluation before starting your exercise program and at regular intervals thereafter.

☐ Find out whether you need direct medical supervision when you exercise—and for what period of time.

☐ Be thoroughly versed in the warning signs of an impending cardiac complication.

☐ Don't exercise in adverse climatic conditions, particularly without taking adequate precautions.

☐ Skip exercise when you have a fever, influenza, or other moderately serious acute illness.

☐ Wear quality shoes designed for the specific type of weight-bearing exercise you are doing.

☐ Don't perform too much exercise too early on in your program.

☐ Know the tell-tale signs of overtraining, and closely monitor your body's response to exercise to make sure you're not overdoing it.

❏ Never disregard a trend indicating that your fatigue or other symptoms are worsening.

❏ Ask your doctor if any medications you're taking require you to take special precautions during exercise.

Appendix A

CFS:
The CDC's Definition

I n an attempt to devise a definition for CFS suitable for use in future research, the CDC organized an informal working group of public health epidemiologists, academic researchers, and clinicians. Their recommendations were published in *Annals of Internal Medicine* in March 1988. Because CFS currently has no diagnostic test, the CDC's definition was based on symptoms and physical signs only, as follows: A case of CFS must fulfill major criteria 1 and 2 (description follows), and the following minor criteria: either a combination of 6 or more of the 11 symptom criteria and 2 or more of the 3 physical criteria, or 8 or more of the 11 symptom criteria.

MAJOR CRITERIA

1. New onset of persistent or relapsing, debilitating fatigue or easy fatigability in a person who has no previous history of similar symptoms that does not resolve with bed rest and that is severe enough to reduce or impair average daily activity below 50% of the person's usual level for a period of at least 6 months

2. Exclusion of the many other clinical conditions that may produce similar symptoms by thorough examination of a medical history, physical examination, and appropriate laboratory testing

MINOR CRITERIA

To fulfill a symptom criterion, a symptom must have begun at or after the time of increased fatigability and must have persisted or recurred over a period of at least 6 months. Individual symptoms may or may not have occurred simultaneously. Physical criteria must be documented by a physician on at least two occasions at least 1 month apart.

Symptom Criteria

1. Mild fever—oral temperature between 99.5 °F (37.5 °C) and 101.5 °F (38.6 °C) when measured by the patient—or chills (Note: Oral temperatures of greater than 101.5 °F [38.6 °C] definitely warrant a search for other causes of illness.)
2. Sore throat
3. Painful lymph nodes in the neck or armpit regions
4. Unexplained generalized muscle weakness
5. Muscle discomfort or pain
6. Prolonged (24 hours or greater) generalized fatigue after levels of exercise that would have been easily tolerated prior to the onset of the illness
7. Generalized headaches of a type, severity, or pattern different from headaches the patients may have had prior to the onset of their illness
8. Arthritis or joint pain that is not accompanied by joint swelling or redness and that appears to shift from one joint to another spontaneously
9. One or more neuropsychological complaints, such as abnormal visual intolerance to light or other transient visual disturbances, forgetfulness, excessive irritability, confusion, difficulty thinking, inability to concentrate, or depression
10. Sleep disturbances—either an inability to sleep (insomnia) or excessive sleeping (hypersomnia)

11. Indication by the patient that the major symptoms initially developed over a few hours or a few days

Physical Criteria

1. Low-grade fever—oral temperature between 99.7 °F (37.6 °C) and 101.5 °F (38.6 °C), or rectal temperature between 100 °F (37.8 °C) and 101.8 °F (38.8 °C) (Note: Higher temperatures than these definitely warrant a further search for the cause of illness.)
2. Inflammation of the pharynx or back of the throat, without evidence of pus in that region
3. Palpable or tender lymph nodes in the neck or armpit regions (Note: Lymph nodes larger than 0.78 inches [2 centimeters] suggest other causes and definitely warrant further evaluation.)

Adapted, with permission, from G.P. Holmes et al., "Chronic Fatigue Syndrome: A Working Case Definition," *Annals of Internal Medicine*, 1988, 108:387-389. Copyright 1988 by American College of Physicians.

Appendix B

How to Take Your Pulse and Calculate Your Heart Rate

Y ou have two pulse points to choose from—the radial artery in your wrist or the carotid artery in your throat. Your radial artery is the preferred place because the reading there is usually more accurate.

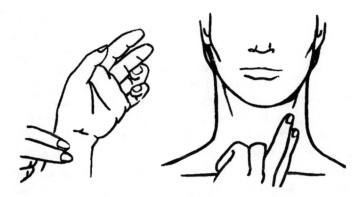

Figure B.1 Pulse points: left) radial artery, right) carotid artery. *Note.* From *ACSM Fitness Book* (p. 24) by The American College of Sports Medicine, 1992, Champaign, IL: Leisure Press. Copyright 1992 by The American College of Sports Medicine. Reprinted by permission.

Your two carotid arteries are located on either side of your windpipe. These arteries are large, and you should be able to locate them easily by gently pressing just to the right or left of your Adam's apple. But there are several things you must keep in mind. Don't press hard; press on only one carotid artery at a time; and do not press too near the jawbone. If you do any of these things your heart rate may slow down excessively and result in potentially harmful consequences, not to mention an inaccurate reading.

Taking your pulse is a three-step process. Here are instructions for taking a wrist pulse reading. Resort to your carotid artery only if you absolutely cannot locate the radial artery in your wrist.

1. *Locate the pulse in your wrist.* The hand of your wristwatch arm is the one you will use to monitor the pulse in your opposite wrist. Your "sensors" are the pads of your fingers, not your fingertips.

Place your index finger and middle finger at the base of the outer third of your wrist, the side on which your thumb is located. If you feel your wrist's tendons, you need to move your fingers further to the outside of your wrist. Do this incrementally, changing the location of your fingers by about a quarter of an inch until you finally locate a pulsation. Don't press too hard or you may obliterate your pulse. A light but firm pressure is all that is needed. You should be able to feel your pulse each time your heart beats, thus making your pulse rate equivalent to your heart rate.

2. *Count your pulse.* To determine your *resting heart rate*, count for 30 to 60 seconds. Your heart rate varies with your breathing; it slows down when you exhale and speeds up when you inhale. Thus if you count your pulse for shorter periods, you won't get a good average reading.

Taking a reading during exercise is different. Then your pulse rate is faster so a 10-second count is sufficient. If you're exercising in a stationary position—on a cycle ergometer, for example—you can count your pulse easily without stopping. However, if you're moving— such as walking or jogging—you'll need to stop, but not completely. Keep your legs moving while you take your pulse, which *you must do immediately*. If you wait for more than a second or two, your heart starts to slow down. This is true particularly if you are fit. If you count for longer than 10 seconds, you run the risk of greatly *underestimating* your heart rate.

When counting your pulse, count as "one" the first pulsation you feel *after* your watchhand hits a digit. Do *not* count as "one" any pulsation that occurs at the same time as the hand hits the digit. Continue the count until your watch registers 10 seconds. If a pulsation occurs at the same time as the watchhand hits the 10-second point, count it, but none thereafter.

3. *Calculate your heart rate.* After you've counted your pulse for 10 seconds, multiply that number by 6 to get your heart rate (beats per minute). Here's a chart with the calculations already done for 10-second pulse counts of 12 through 31:

12 = 72	17 = 102	22 = 132	27 = 162
13 = 78	18 = 108	23 = 138	28 = 168
14 = 84	19 = 114	24 = 144	29 = 174
15 = 90	20 = 120	25 = 150	30 = 180
16 = 96	21 = 126	26 = 156	31 = 186

Appendix C

Tests and Procedures in a Thorough Pre-Exercise Medical Exam

Below, I describe what happens during a state-of-the-art medical exam in a facility that's fully equipped for sophisticated testing. Your checkup may not be as comprehensive if the equipment isn't available or if your medical history indicates that your case simply doesn't warrant it.

 Checkup Checklist

_____ My physician or physician's assistant takes a thorough medical history to identify the diseases I know I have or any symptoms suggestive of disease, and to document all the medications I'm currently taking. It also covers my attitudes about exercise and CFS in general, and my ability to perform the physical activities of daily living.

I'm examined for other illnesses. In particular, I'm given a thorough cardiovascular exam, which includes

_____ blood pressure measurement

_____ monitoring of the pulses in my neck, arms, and legs

_____ listening to my neck, chest, heart, abdomen, and femoral arteries in my groin with a stethoscope

_____ inspection of the veins in my neck, examination of my abdomen, and inspection of my ankles for any evidence of heart failure

_____ a blood-cholesterol test, if none has been done recently. If the result this time is 200 mg/dl (5.17 mmol/L) or higher, a more detailed blood-lipid profile is ordered showing the ratio of the so-called good HDL-cholesterol to the bad LDL-cholesterol.

_____ a resting electrocardiogram (ECG)

_____ a treadmill exercise test—known as a "symptom-limited maximal exercise test"—with ECG and blood pressure monitoring. This test is especially important if any of these conditions apply:

- My CFS followed an acute viral or flu-like illness;
- I am severely impaired or debilitated by my CFS (see chapter 2);
- I have two or more major coronary artery disease risk factors:

  - high blood pressure
  - a blood-cholesterol level above 239 mg/dl or 6.18 mmol/L
  - cigarette smoking
  - diabetes
  - a family history of coronary artery disease or other atherosclerotic disease

- I have any known or suspected cardiovascular disease;
- I have known or suspected lung disease;
- I'm a man over 40 years old;
- I'm a woman over 50 years old.

For any person with one or more of these conditions who is about to embark on an aerobic exercise program, this is the precautionary approach strongly recommended by the American College of Sports Medicine (ACSM). While the ACSM has no specific recommendations for CFS patients, they do recommend that people with "unaccustomed short-ness of breath or shortness of breath with mild exertion" have an exercise test.

_____ I'm checked out for musculoskeletal problems that may limit my ability to exercise or that may be worsened by exercise.

_____ My abdomen is examined, particularly to determine if my spleen is enlarged.

_____ My body weight and, if possible, percentage body fat are measured.

_____ My physician reviews the results of all pertinent tests that have been performed on me in the past.

_____ My physician uses his or her judgment in deciding what additional tests I need given my individual circumstances and taking into consideration the various clinical and laboratory tests recommended by the CDC (published in the March 1988 issue of _Annals of Internal Medicine_) for persons who suffer from unexplained chronic fatigue.

Notes

FOREWORD

[1]Chen, M.K. "The Epidemiology of Self-Perceived Fatigue Among Adults." *Preventive Medicine* 15 (1986): 74-81.

[2]U.S. Department of Health and Human Services. "The National Ambulatory Medical Care Survey." *Vital and Health Statistics*, Series 13, No. 93, 1988.

CHAPTER 1

[1]Eichner, E.R. "Chronic Fatigue Syndrome: Searching for the Cause and Treatment." *Physician and Sportsmedicine* 17 (1989): 142-152.

[2]Rush, A.J. "Problems Associated With the Diagnosis of Depression." *Journal of Clinical Psychiatry* 15 (1990): 15-22.

[3]Holmes, G.P., et al. "Chronic Fatigue Syndrome: A Working Case Definition." *Annals of Internal Medicine* 108 (1988): 387-389.

[4]Kroenke, K., et al. "Chronic Fatigue in Primary Care." *Journal of the American Medical Association* 260 (1988): 929-934.

[5]Gold, D., et al. "Chronic Fatigue, A Prospective Clinic and Virologic Study." *Journal of the American Medical Association* 264 (1990): 48-53.

[6]Beard, G. *American Nervousness*. New York: G.P. Putnam's, 1881.

[7]Acheson, E.D. "The Clinical Syndrome Variously Called Benign Myalgic Encephalomyelitis, Iceland Disease and Epidemic Neuromyasthenia." *American Journal of Medicine* April (1959): 569-595.

[8]Oldstone, M.B. "Viral Persistence and Immune Dysfunction." *Hospital Practice* May (1990): 81-98.

[9]DeFreitas, E., et al. "Retroviral Sequences Related to Human T-Lymphotropic Virus Type II in Patients with Chronic Fatigue Immune Dysfunction Syndrome." *Proceedings of the National Academy of Science* 88 (1991): 2922-2926.

[10]Shafran, S.D. "The Chronic Fatigue Syndrome." *American Journal of Medicine* 90 (1991): 730-739.

[11]Straus, S.E., et al. "Allergy and the Chronic Fatigue Syndrome." *Journal of Allergy and Clinical Immunology* May (1988): 791-795.

[12]Lloyd, A., et al. "A Double-Blind Placebo-Controlled Trial of Intravenous Immunoglobulin Therapy in Patients with Chronic Fatigue Syndrome." *American Journal of Medicine* 89 (1990): 561-568.

[13]Feiden, K. *Hope and Help for Chronic Fatigue Syndrome.* New York: Prentice Hall Press, 1990.

[14]Petty, F. "Southwestern Internal Medicine Conference: Depression and Medical Illness." *American Journal of the Medical Sciences* 296 (1989): 59-68.

[15]Greenberg, D.B. "Neurasthenia in the 1980s: Chronic Mononucleosis, Chronic Fatigue Syndrome, and Anxiety and Depressive Disorders." *Psychosomatics* 31 (1990): 129-137.

[16]Stricklin, A., Sewell, M., and Austad, C. "Objective Measurement of Personality Variables in Epidemic Neuromyasthenia Patients." *South African Medical Journal* 77 (1990): 31-34.

[17]Ray, C. "Chronic Fatigue Syndrome and Depression: Conceptual and Methodological Ambiguities." *Psychological Medicine* 21 (1991): 1-9.

[18]Daruna, J.H., and Margan, J.E. "Psychosocial Effects on Immune Function: Neuroendocrine Pathways." *Psychosomatics* 31 (1990): 4-12.

[19]Feiden, K. *Hope and Help for Chronic Fatigue Syndrome.* New York: Prentice Hall Press, 1990.

[20]Lloyd, A.R. "Muscle Versus Brain: Chronic Fatigue Syndrome." *Medical Journal of Australia* 153 (1990): 530-534.

CHAPTER 2

[1]Leon, A.S., et al. "Leisure-Time Physical Activity Levels and Risk of Coronary Heart Disease and Death." *Journal of the American Medical Association* 248 (1987): 2388-2395.

[2]Fisher, G.C. *Chronic Fatigue Syndrome.* New York: Warner Books, 1989.

[3]Bouchard, C., et al. (eds.). *Exercise, Fitness, and Health. A Consensus of Current Knowledge.* Champaign, IL: Human Kinetics Publishers, 1990.

[4]Centers for Disease Control. "Coronary Heart Disease Attributable to Sedentary Lifestyle — Selected States, 1988." *Journal of the American Medical Association* 19 (1990): 1390-1392.

[5]Powell, K.E., et al. "Physical Activity and the Incidence of Coronary Heart Disease." *Annual Review of Public Health* 8 (1987): 253-287.

[6]Berlin, G.A., and Colditz, G.A. "A Meta-Analysis of Physical Activity in the Prevention of Coronary Heart Disease." *American Journal of Epidemiology* 132 (1990): 612-628.

[7]Buchwald, D., et al. "Frequency of 'Chronic Active Epstein-Barr Virus Infection' in a General Medical Practice." *Journal of the American Medical Association* 257 (1987): 2303-2307.

[8]Lewis, S.F., and Haller, R.G. "Physiologic Measurement of Exercise and Fatigue with Special Reference to Chronic Fatigue Syndrome." *Reviews of Infectious Diseases* 13 (1991): S98-S108.

[9]Lloyd, A.R. "Muscle Versus Brain: Chronic Fatigue Syndrome." *Medical Journal of Australia* 153 (1990): 530-534.

[10]Montague, T.J., et al. "Cardiac Function at Rest and With Exercise in the Chronic Fatigue Syndrome." *Chest* 95 (1989): 779-784.

[11]Kottke, F.J. "The Effects of Limitation of Activity Upon the Human Body." *Journal of the American Medical Association* 196 (1966): 825-830.

[12]Saltin, B., et al. "Response to Exercise After Bed Rest and After Training." *Circulation* 38 (1968): VII-1–VII-78.

[13]Edwards, R.H.T. "Muscle Fatigue and Pain." *Acta Medica Scandinavica Supplementum* 711 (1986): 179-188.

[14]Holmgren, A., et al. "Physical Training of Patients with Vasoregulatory Asthenia." *Acta Medica Scandinavica* 158 (1957): 436-446.

[15]Kohl, H.W., Moorefield, D.L., and Blair, S.N. "Is Cardiorespiratory Fitness Associated with General Chronic Fatigue in Apparently Healthy Men and Women?" *Medicine and Science in Sports and Exercise* 19 (1987): S6.

[16]Goldenberg, D.L., et al. "High Frequency of Fibromyalgia in Patients with Chronic Fatigue Syndrome Seen in Primary Care Practice." *Arthritis and Rheumatism* 33 (1990): 381-387.

[17]McCain, G.A., et al. "A Controlled Study of the Effects of a Supervised Cardiovascular Fitness Training Program on the Manifestations of Primary Fibromyalgia." *Arthritis and Rheumatism* 31 (1988): 1135-1141.

[18]Raglin, G.S. "Exercise and Mental Health. Beneficial and Detrimental Effects." *Sports Medicine* 9 (1990): 323-329.

[19]Sidney, K.H., and Jerome, W.C. "Anxiety and Depression: Exercise for Mood Enhancement." In *Current Therapy in Sports Medicine-2*, edited by J.S. Torg et al. Toronto: B.C. Decker, Inc., 1990.

[20]Thoren, P., et al. "Endorphins and Exercise: Physiological Mechanisms and Clinical Implications." *Medicine and Science in Sports and Exercise* 22 (1990): 417-428.

[21]Macera, C., et al. "Predicting Lower-Extremity Injuries Among Habitual Runners." *Archives of Internal Medicine* 149 (1989): 2565-2568.

[22]Walter, S., et al. "The Ontario Cohort Study of Running-Related Injuries." *Archives of Internal Medicine* 149 (1989): 2561-2564.

[23]Blair, S.N., Kohl, H.W., and Goodyear, N.N. "Rates and Risks for Running and Exercise Injuries: Studies in Three Populations." *Research Quarterly for Exercise and Sport* 58 (1987): 221-228.

[24]Thompson, P.D., et al. "Incidence of Death During Jogging in Rhode Island From 1975 Through 1980." *Journal of the American Medical Association* 247 (1982): 2535-2538.

[25]Gordon, N.F., and Gibbons, L.W. *The Cooper Clinic Cardiac Rehabilitation Program.* New York: Simon & Schuster, 1990.

[26]Montague, T.J., et al. "Cardiac Function at Rest and With Exercise in the Chronic Fatigue Syndrome." *Chest* 95 (1989): 779-781.

[27]Gatmaitan, B.G., Chason, J.L., and Lerner, A.M. "Augmentation of the Virulence of Murine Coxsackie-Virus B-3 Myocardiopathy by Exercise." *Journal of Experimental Medicine* 131 (1970): 1120-1136.

[28]Ilback, N.G., Fohlman, J., and Friman, G. "Exercise in Coxsackie B3 Myocarditis: Effects on Heart Lymphocyte Subpopulations and the Inflammatory Reaction." *American Heart Journal* 117 (1989): 1298-1302.

[29]Calabrese, L.H. "Exercise, Immunity, Cancer, and Infection." In *Exercise, Fitness, and Health. A Consensus of Current Knowledge*, edited by C. Bouchard et al. Champaign, IL: Human Kinetics Publishers, 1990.

[30]Dalrymple, W. "Infectious Mononucleosis: Relation of Bed Rest and Activity to Prognosis." *Postgraduate Medicine* 35 (1964): 345-349.

[31]Simon, H.B. "Discussion: Exercise, Immunity, Cancer, and Infection," In *Exercise, Fitness, and Health. A Consensus of Current Knowledge*, edited by C. Bouchard et al. Champaign, IL: Human Kinetics Publishers, 1990.

[32]Wessely, S. "Old Wine in New Bottles: Neurasthenia and 'ME'." *Psychological Medicine* 20 (1990): 35-53.

[33]Smith, J., et al. "Exercise Training and Neutrophil Microbicidal Activity." *International Journal of Sports Medicine* 11 (1990): 179-187.

CHAPTER 3

[1]Institute for Aerobics Research. *The Strength Connection.* Dallas: Institute for Aerobics Research, 1990.

[2]American College of Sports Medicine. "Position Stand. The Recommended Quantity and Quality of Exercise for Developing and Maintaining Cardiorespiratory Fitness and Muscular Fitness in Healthy Adults." *Medicine and Science in Sports and Exercise* 22 (1990): 265-274.

[3]Gordon, N.F., and Gibbons, L.W. *The Cooper Clinic Cardiac Rehabilitation Program.* New York: Simon & Schuster, 1990.

[4]Agre, J.C., et al. "Light Resistance and Stretching Exercise in Elderly Women: Effect Upon Strength." *Archives of Physical Medicine and Rehabilitation* 69 (1988): 273-276.

[5]Cooper, K.H. *Aerobics.* New York: Bantam Books, 1968.

[6]Blair, S.N., et al. "Exercise and Fitness in Childhood: Implications for a Lifetime of Health." In *Perspectives in Exercise Science and Sports Medicine*, edited by C.V. Gisolfi and D.R. Lamb. Vol. 2: *Youth, Exercise and Sport*. Indianapolis: Benchmark Press, 1989, pp. 401-430.

[7]American Heart Association Medical/Scientific Statement. "Exercise Standards. A Statement for Health Professionals From the American Heart Association." *Circulation* 82 (1990): 2286-2322.

[8]Haskell, W.L., Montoye, H.J., and Orenstein, D. "Physical Activity and Exercise to Achieve Health-Related Physical Fitness Components." *Public Health Reports* 100 (1985): 202-212.

[9]Blair, S.N. *Living with Exercise*. Dallas: American Health Publishing Company, 1991.

[10]DeBusk, R.F., et al. "Training Effects of Long Versus Short Bouts of Exercise in Healthy Subjects." *American Journal of Cardiology* 65 (1990): 1010-1013.

[11]Brill, P.A., et al. "The Effect of Chronic Fatigue on the Physiological Response to Graded Exercise Testing." *Medicine and Science in Sports and Exercise* 23 (1991): S166.

[12]Stokes, M.J., Cooper, R.G., and Edwards, R.H.T. "Normal Muscle Strength and Fatigability in Patients with Effort Syndromes." *British Medical Journal* 279 (1988): 1014-1016.

[13]Montague, T.J., et al. "Cardiac Function at Rest and With Exercise in the Chronic Fatigue Syndrome." *Chest* 95 (1989): 779-784.

[14]American College of Sports Medicine. "Position Stand. The Recommended Quantity and Quality of Exercise for Developing and Maintaining Cardiorespiratory and Muscular Fitness in Healthy Adults." *Medicine and Science in Sports and Exercise* 22 (1990): 265-274.

[15]American College of Sports Medicine. *Guidelines for Exercise Testing and Prescription*. Philadelphia: Lea & Febiger, 1991.

[16]Borg, G.A. "Psychophysical Bases of Perceived Exertion." *Medicine and Science in Sports and Exercise* 14 (1982): 377-387.

[17]Edwards, R.H.T. "Muscle Fatigue and Pain." *Acta Medica Scandinavica Supplementum* 711 (1986): 179-188.

[18]Rippe, J.M., et al. "Walking for Health and Fitness." *Journal of the American Medical Association* 259 (1988): 2720-2724.

[19]Thomas, T.R., and Londeree, B.R. "Energy Cost During Prolonged Walking Vs. Jogging Exercise." *Physician and Sportsmedicine* 17 (1989): 93-102.

CHAPTER 4

[1]Cooper, K.H. *The Aerobics Program for Total Well-Being*. New York: Bantam Books, 1982.

[2]Gwinup, G. "Weight Loss Without Dietary Restriction: Efficacy of Different Forms of Aerobic Exercise." *American Journal of Sports Medicine* 15 (1987): 275-279.

[3]Cooper, K.H. *Overcoming Hypertension*. New York: Bantam Books, 1990.

[4]Cooper, K.H. *The Aerobics Program for Total Well-Being*. New York: Bantam Books, 1982.

[5]DeBenedette, V. "Stair Machines: The Truth About This Fitness Fad." *Physician and Sportsmedicine* 18 (1990): 131-134.

[6]Bartlett, J., et al. "Analysis of the Acute Physiologic Effects of Minitrampoline Rebounding Exercise." *Journal of Cardiopulmonary Rehabilitation* 10 (1990): 395-400.

[7]Williams, C., and Gordon, N. "Bench Stepping." *Shape* April 1990: 96-101.

[8]Gordon, N.F., et al. "Effects of Rest Interval Duration on Cardiorespiratory Responses to Hydraulic Resistance Circuit Training." *Journal of Cardiopulmonary Rehabilitation* 9 (1989): 325-330.

[9]Paffenbarger, R.S., Jr., et al. "Physical Activity, All-Cause Mortality, and Longevity in College Alumni." *New England Journal of Medicine* 314 (1986): 605-613.

[10]Coyle, E.F. "Detraining and Retention of Training-Induced Adaptations." In *Resource Manual for Guidelines for Exercise Testing and Prescription*, edited by S.N. Blair et al. Philadelphia: Lea & Febiger, 1988.

CHAPTER 5

[1]Cooper, K.H. *Running Without Fear*. New York: M. Evans and Co., 1985.

[2]Cooper, K.H. *The Aerobics Program for Total Well-Being*. New York, Bantam Books, 1982.

[3]Cooper, K.H., and Cooper, M. *The New Aerobics for Women*. New York, Bantam Books, 1988.

[4]Holmes, G.P., et al. "Chronic Fatigue Syndrome: A Working Case Definition." *Annals of Internal Medicine* 108 (1988): 387-389.

[5]American College of Sports Medicine. *Guidelines for Exercise Testing and Prescription*. Philadelphia: Lea & Febiger, 1991.

[6]Montague, T.J., et al. "Cardiac Function at Rest and With Exercise in the Chronic Fatigue Syndrome." *Chest* 95 (1989): 779-784.

[7]Thornton, J.S. "Common Concerns About the Common Cold." *Physician and Sportsmedicine* 18 (1990): 120-126.

[8]Levin, S. "Overtraining Causes Olympic-Sized Problems." *Physician and Sportsmedicine* 19 (1991): 112-118.

[9]Noakes, T. *Lore of Running*. Champaign, IL: Leisure Press, 1991.

[10]Clarkson, P. "Too Much Too Soon: The Aftermath of Overexertion." *Gatorade Sports Science Exchange* 21 (January 1990).

[11]Ebbeling, C.B., and Clarkson, P. "Exercise-Induced Muscle Damage and Adaptation." *Sports Medicine* 7 (1989): 207-234.

[12]The Rand Index of Vitality is adapted from R.H. Brook et al., "Overview of Adult Health Status Measures Fielded in Rand's Health Insurance Study." *Medical Care* 17 (1979): 1-55.

Index